C3

To Isobel x

Hap[illegible]

and lots of [illegible]e

from

Rodger x Margaret

x x x

26.9.70.

Cardio-vascular Surgery
For Nurses and Students

Cardio-vascular Surgery For Nurses and Students

William H. Bain,
M.D., F.R.C.S. (Edin. & Glasg.)
Senior Lecturer in Cardio-vascular Surgery
University of Glasgow
Consultant Cardiac Surgeon to Glasgow Royal Infirmary and Stobhill General Hospital

J. Kennedy Watt,
B.Sc., Ch.M., F.R.C.S., F.R.C.S. (Glasg.)
Consultant Surgeon to Glasgow Royal Infirmary and the Peripheral Vascular Unit,
Belvidere Hospital

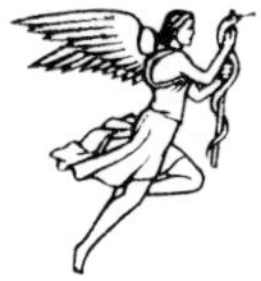

E & S LIVINGSTONE
EDINBURGH AND LONDON, 1970

ISBN 0 443 00709 8

Printed in Great Britain

Preface

The dramatic advances which have occurred in medicine in the past 20 years are nowhere more spectacular than in the field of cardio-vascular surgery, culminating in transplantation of the heart in 1968. Over the years, earlier techniques have been consolidated and new fields are constantly being explored. These achievements have been made possible by advances in ancillary fields—in radiology, which serves to delineate the lesion, in the development of cardiac catheterisation techniques which led to the pacemaker, in anaesthesia and the development of heart-lung bypass techniques, in biochemistry, antibiotics, etc. All these have contributed and have stimulated the surgeon to repair or replace damaged parts so that many people enjoy better and longer lives than formerly.

However dazzling these advances, one must always remember that the surgeon is dealing with diseased or congenitally malformed organs and that he can improve only the mechanics of disease but not the disease itself. The really spectacular advances will come when the incidence of congenital defects can be controlled and when the ravages of rheumatic heart disease and atherosclerosis can be eliminated.

The rapidity of change is such that a textbook becomes rapidly out of date, yet enough time has elapsed and a sufficient number of techniques have become stabilised for our present knowledge to be consolidated in a book such as this.

The book explains in simple terms the basic knowledge and techniques of cardio-vascular surgery. While it has been written primarily for the staff-nurse who wishes to increase her knowledge of this specialised branch of surgery, it is hoped that it will prove useful to all those who wish to acquire a basic knowledge of cardio-vascular surgery.

The authors wish to acknowledge the invaluable collaboration of Miss Jean McDonald, D.A. (Glasg.), A.I.M.I., medical artist, who was responsible for the illustrations, Mr W. E. Towler, for the photographic work, and Miss Margaret Black and Mrs Mary Baird, who typed the manuscript. We are also grateful to those who read and criticised the draft manuscript. Figure 28 is reproduced by courtesy of Dr J. A. Kennedy, Department of Medical Cardiology, Figure 40 by courtesy of Dr W. Duguid, Department of Pathology and Figures 59 and 60 by courtesy of Dr J. D. Briggs, Renal Dialysis Unit, all of Glasgow Royal Infirmary.

Finally, we take this opportunity of acknowledging our indebtedness to the members of the nursing staff who have worked in the wards and intensive care areas over the years.

Glasgow, 1970

W. H. Bain
J. K. Watt

Contents

CHAPTER 1

Anatomy and Physiology of the Heart

The heart lies in the centre of the mediastinum with its apex downwards and to the left. Anteriorly, it is protected by the sternum and costal cartilages and, posteriorly, it is related to the oesophagus and main bronchi. On each side it is cushioned by the lungs. It rests on the diaphragm below and from its upper surface the principal arteries arch upwards. The heart is enclosed in a sac of fibrous tissue, the pericardium, whose endothelial surfaces move freely over each other and permit contraction and relaxation with relatively little friction.

Anatomically and functionally, the heart is divided into right

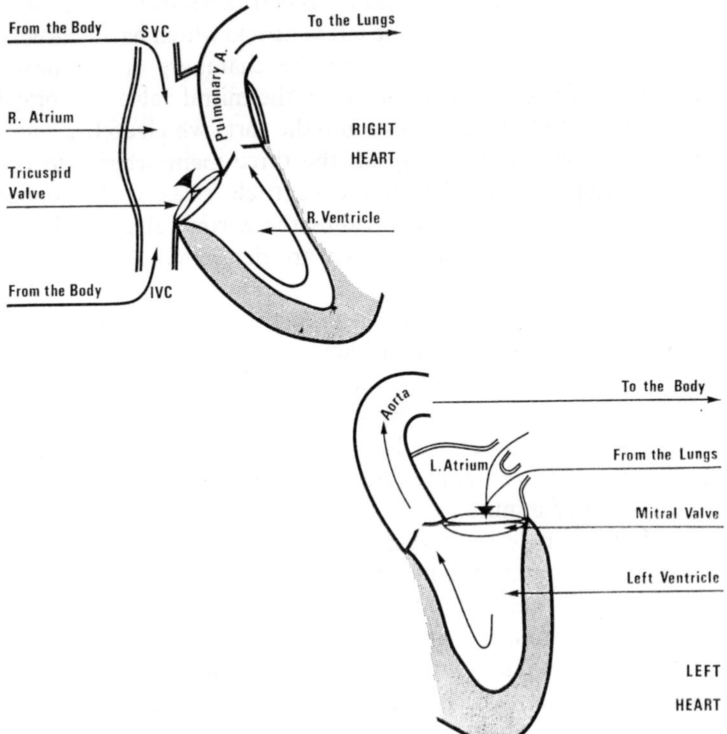

FIG. 1. The right and left halves of the heart.

and left halves, each of which is constructed to the same basic pattern (Fig. 1).

The right heart consists of the superior and inferior venae cavae, the right atrium, right ventricle and pulmonary artery and it pumps venous blood from the body through the pulmonary circulation. There are two non-return valves at the inlet and outlet of the ventricle—the tricuspid valve between the atrium and ventricle and the pulmonary valve between the ventricle and pulmonary artery. The atrium functions mainly as a collecting chamber with very little contractile power and the ventricle supplies the power necessary to send blood through the pulmonary circulation to the left side of the heart.

The left heart pumps the blood which has been oxygenated in the lungs through the rest of the body—the systemic circulation. It comprises the pulmonary veins (two on each side), the left atrium and ventricle, and the aorta. Blood flows from the atrium through the mitral valve into the left ventricle which has the thickest and most muscular wall of all the chambers of the heart. Contraction of the left ventricle closes the mitral valve and blood is forced through the aortic valve into the aorta which arches backwards then downwards giving off the three main arteries to the head and upper limbs. When the ventricle relaxes, the higher pressure of blood in the aorta closes the aortic valve and blood flows into the right and left coronary arteries which arise immediately beyond the aortic valve.

Both halves of the heart contract simultaneously and each pumps out exactly the same volume of blood because any discrepancy in output would lead to engorgement of either the pulmonary or systemic circulations. The output of either ventricle is called the *cardiac output* and, when the body is at rest, this is approximately 5 litres of blood per minute (3·2 litres per square metre of body surface area per minute).

The left ventricle has to generate a relatively high pressure to propel blood through the many channels of the systemic circulation. The right ventricle has the easier task of pumping blood through the pulmonary circulation. It is therefore less muscular and a lower pulmonary arterial pressure is sufficient to ensure an adequate flow rate. The left ventricle is the more muscular of the two pumping chambers and normal pressures in the left heart are higher than in the right heart (Fig. 2).

Arterial pressure is controlled by a neuro-humoral system of regulators including the carotid sinus situated at the bifurcation of the common carotid artery, the secretion of vasopressor substances by the kidney and the secretion of adrenaline by the adrenal medulla. In general, an increase in the peripheral resistance of either the pulmonary or systemic circulations demands a higher arterial pressure to force blood through the circuit and the ventricle has to increase its force of contraction.

The pressure in the systemic arteries is maintained by the left ventricle which adjusts its output and force according to the resistance to flow offered by the smallest arteries (arterioles) and capillaries. The arterioles have muscular walls which relax (vasodilatation) or contract (vasoconstriction) in response to different circumstances. By dilatation of some arterioles and constriction of others, blood can be diverted to wherever the need for blood is greatest. For example, after a meal a large volume of blood must flow through the vessels of the stomach, intestines and liver so as to deal with the products of digestion. The intestinal arterioles therefore dilate and receive an increased blood flow and, at the same time, arterioles in the muscles of the arms and legs are constricted and receive less blood. If extra blood flow is required in several parts of the body at the same time, the left ventricle must

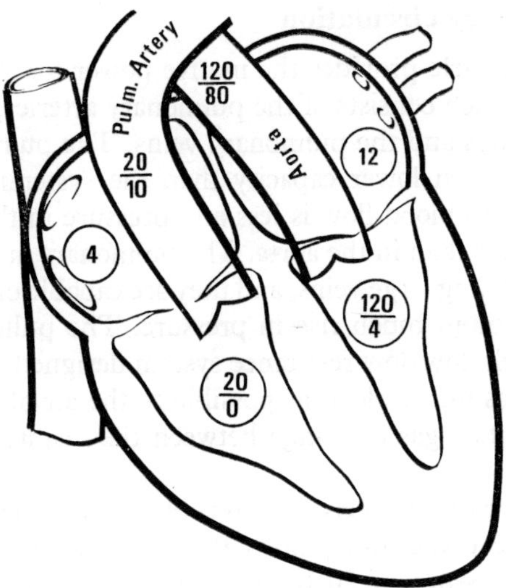

FIG. 2. The normal intra-cardiac pressures.

increase its output and the stroke volume (the amount of blood pumped out with each contraction) and the heart rate are increased. The diversion of blood from skeletal muscle to intestine which occurs after a meal is the reason why one is advised not to indulge in strenuous muscular activity after eating.

If all the arterioles in the body dilate simultaneously, the blood pressure in the main arteries can fall to dangerously low levels, as occurs in 'shock' due to bacterial toxaemia. On the other hand, drugs which produce a moderate degree of arteriolar dilatation can be useful in the treatment of patients with hypertension. Conversely, patients with low blood pressure can be given vasopressor drugs, e.g., noradrenaline (Levophed), which cause constriction of arterioles and raise the blood pressure.

Maintenance of a normal blood pressure is ultimately dependent on the strength of the left ventricular pump and, if this fails, blood pressure falls no matter what the arterioles do. In coronary thrombosis, the blockage of a coronary artery deprives part of the myocardium of its blood supply and that area of muscle dies and becomes an infarct. The arterioles become constricted in an effort to maintain blood pressure, but this resistance increases the work load of the left ventricle, which may fail to maintain an adequate circulation and the patient dies.

The pulmonary circulation

The right ventricle provides the motive power for the pulmonary circulation, which consists of the pulmonary arteries, the capillary bed of the lungs and the pulmonary veins. The pulmonary circulation has a much lower capacity than the systemic circulation, the resistance to blood flow is less and pressure in the pulmonary arteries is lower than in the aorta. The pulmonary arteries are thin walled, resembling large veins, and they are capable of considerable distension without much rise in pressure. The pulmonary circulation is a high flow–low resistance system designed in such a way as to expose as much blood as possible to the air of the alveoli in order to facilitate gas exchange between the inspired air and the blood.

The right ventricle receives venous blood from the superior and inferior venae cavae and pumps this into the main pulmonary artery at a pressure of 20/10 mm. Hg. The pulmonary artery, which is the same size as the aorta, divides into two about 5 cm.

above the heart. Within each lung these arteries divide further to supply each lobe, splitting up into smaller and smaller branches which ultimately form the network of capillaries around the alveoli. In the alveoli, the blood in the capillaries is separated from the air by only two layers of cells—the capillary endothelium and the alveolar lining—and oxygen and carbon dioxide can diffuse readily through these cells. Beyond the alveoli, the capillaries join to form venules which return blood to the pulmonary veins which transport the newly oxygenated blood to the left atrium.

The coronary circulation

The myocardium requires a liberal blood supply to satisfy its oxygen needs and to carry away the waste products of its metabolism because it must work continuously, without any rest other than that occurring during muscular relaxation in diastole. In the adult, the coronary circulation requires from 300 to 500 ml. per minute of blood at rest.

The coronary arteries are the first branches of the aorta. They arise at the level of the cusps of the aortic valve and run round the heart in the groove between the atria and ventricles. The important left anterior descending coronary artery arises from the left coronary artery just beyond its origin and runs down the front of the heart between the right and left ventricles to reach the apex. The other main branch of the left coronary artery is called the circumflex and it follows the left atrio-ventricular groove to end on the postero-inferior surface of the heart.

The right coronary artery arises from the front of the aorta and runs in the right atrio-ventricular groove. It terminates on the postero-inferior surface of the heart, by anastomosing with the branches of the left coronary artery.

The coronary veins accompany the arteries and join to form one large vein (the coronary sinus) which empties into the right atrium just above the tricuspid valve.

The circulation before birth

A knowledge of the anatomy of the heart and circulation of the foetus (Fig. 3) is essential to the understanding of many forms of congenital heart disease.

In utero, the baby's blood is oxygenated by the placenta. The lungs are collapsed and airless until breathing commences after

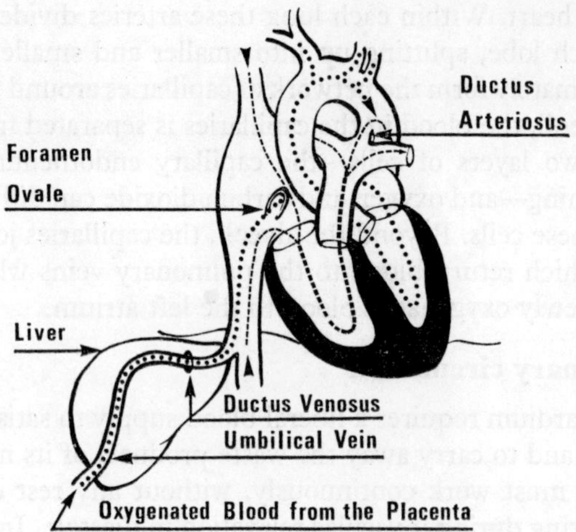

FIG. 3. The foetal circulation: the dotted line represents oxygenated blood; the dashed line deoxygenated blood.

birth and only a minimum blood supply is required at this time.

Oxygenated blood flows along the umbilical vein to the ductus venosus which bypasses the liver and joins the inferior vena cava. This blood enters the right atrium and passes through an opening in the inter-atrial septum (foramen ovale) to the left atrium and the left ventricle pumps it through the systemic circulation.

The superior vena cava carries venous blood from the head, neck and arms to the right atrium, and this stream of blood flows through the tricuspid valve into the right ventricle. The right ventricle pumps this blood into the pulmonary artery and it bypasses the lungs by going through the ductus arteriosus into the aorta where it joins the outflow from the left ventricle.

Shortly after the baby is born, the ductus venosus, the foramen ovale and the ductus arteriosus close. If either of the latter two do not close, the child will be born with an interatrial septal defect (foramen ovale type) or a patent ductus arteriosus.

CHAPTER 2

Haemodynamic Principles and Symptomatology in Heart Disease

Haemodynamic Principles

When the heart is diseased or congenitally abnormal, compensatory changes occur in the heart and circulation in order to maintain function. These compensatory changes can be recognised clinically and may provide diagnostic clues but in some cases symptoms do not arise until the compensatory mechanisms have failed.

The heart and lungs, the arteries and veins all require to adapt to the altered mechanics of disease and the degree of adaptation varies according to whether the lesion is a septal defect, a valvular or other type of stenosis, or a valvular incompetence.

Septal defects

A 'hole in the heart' (a defect in either the atrial or ventricular septum), or a patent ductus arteriosus results in the abnormal shunt of blood from one side of the heart to the other. The direction of flow through the defect depends on the difference in blood pressure between the two chambers connected by the hole. Study of the cardiac pressures (Fig. 2) shows that the pressures in the left heart and aorta are higher than in the right heart and pulmonary artery. Blood therefore flows from left to right through an atrial septal defect, a ventricular septal defect, or a patent ductus arteriosus.

These left to right shunts increase the amount of blood flowing through the pulmonary circulation, and the right heart and pulmonary artery have to cope with the normal venous return from the venae cavae, plus the additional arterial blood flowing through the shunt.

Consequently, the pulmonary circulation is constantly overfilled with blood. If excessive pulmonary flow continues for many years, the small blood vessels of the lung develop thickening of their walls and narrowing of the lumen and this increases the resistance to blood flow through the pulmonary circulation. The right ventricle hypertrophies to deal with the increased arteriolar resistance and the additional flow coming through the shunt, and blood pressure rises in the main pulmonary arteries (pulmonary hypertension). Eventually, the changes in the pulmonary vessels become irreversible and present surgical techniques are unable to improve the patient's symptoms. If the shunt is small and the right heart is able to compensate, symptoms may be few. If the shunt is a large one, overfilling of the lungs gives rise to dyspnoea, haemoptysis and signs of right ventricular hypertrophy. Sooner or later, the right ventricle is unable to carry the extra load and right heart failure ensues. This results in engorgement of the systemic venous circulation which is recognised clinically by jugular vein distension, liver enlargement and ankle oedema.

Valvular stenosis

In common with other organs and muscles of the body, the heart responds to an increase in work load by hypertrophy (an increase in muscle bulk, capacity, and force of contraction) and to a decrease in work by atrophy (a decrease in size and force of contraction). This fundamental principle is an important guide to the understanding and diagnosis of heart disease.

For example, when a patient develops aortic stenosis as a result of rheumatic fever in childhood, the aortic valve leaflets stick together and the orifice becomes narrowed. The left ventricle has to work harder to pump blood through the stenosis into the aorta, and it becomes more and more muscular. This hypertrophy produces signs which form the diagnostic clues in aortic stenosis. The apex beat becomes more powerful, more easily palpable, and more sustained than normal and the ECG pattern alters in a characteristic manner as a larger electrical impulse is generated (Appendix A). The X-ray silhouette of the heart may show a bulge corresponding to the enlarged left ventricle but, with outflow valve stenosis, the ventricle usually enlarges inwards at the expense of the cavity, and only extreme degrees of hypertrophy are seen on a straight X-ray.

In mitral stenosis, the valve between the left atrium and ventricle is narrowed. The first chamber to be overworked is the left atrium which becomes larger and thick-walled. However, the ventricles are mainly responsible for providing the pumping forces which circulate the blood and Figure 4 shows that it is the right ventricle which really pushes the blood through the mitral valve,

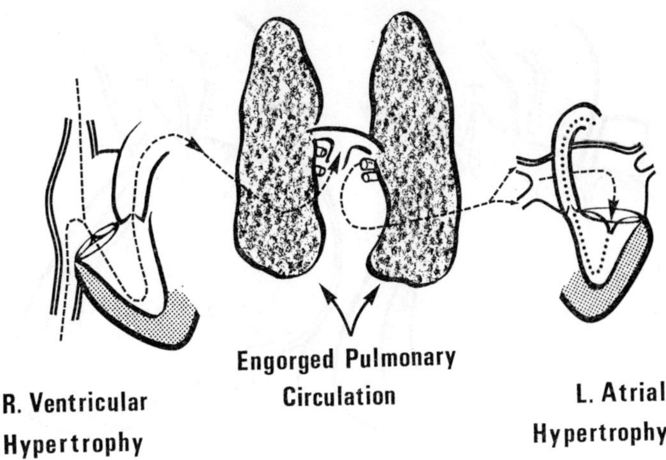

FIG. 4. The haemodynamic consequences of mitral stenosis.

having first pumped it through the lungs. Consequently, patients with mitral stenosis develop hypertrophy of the right ventricle. This can be felt heaving to the left of the sternum and the ECG often shows a characteristic diagnostic pattern of right ventricular preponderance (Appendix A). The left ventricle receives less blood than normal and becomes smaller and less muscular.

Extreme degrees of ventricular hypertrophy are seen in patients who have survived into adult life despite congenital stenosis of the aortic or pulmonary valves. After operative correction of the valvular stenosis in these patients, the excessively muscular walls of the ventricle tend to meet during systole and constitute a continuing obstruction particularly in the region of the outflow tract (Fig. 5). In the early post-operative period the output per beat (stroke volume) from such a ventricle is exceedingly small, and an adequate cardiac output is dependent on a fast heart rate. Surgery in these patients carries a high mortality risk, and the post-operative period is characterised by a dangerously low cardiac output for several days. Fortunately, atrophy of the myocardium occurs with the passage of time and, if the patient survives the critical first post-operative week, a satisfactory end result can be anticipated.

Valvular incompetence

When one of the heart valves is incompetent, a proportion of each

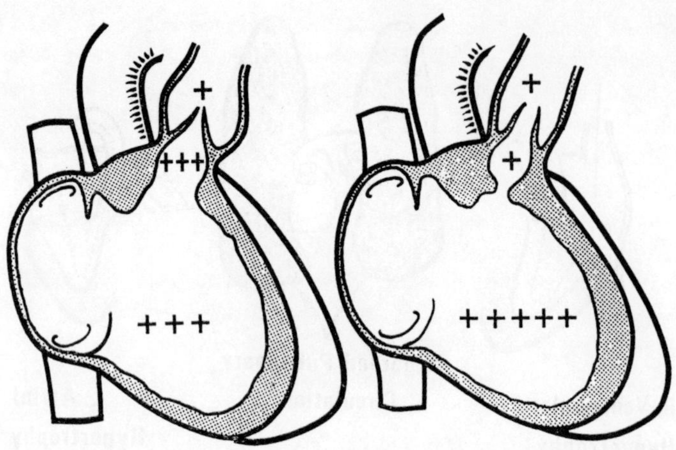

FIG. 5. 'Suicidal right ventricle'. The drawing demonstrates how the excessively hypertrophied outflow tract of the right ventricle may obstruct blood flow after relief of pulmonary valvular stenosis. (R. Brock, 1957. *The Anatomy of Congenital Pulmonary Stenosis*, London: Cassell.)

stroke volume leaks back during diastole. This results in a net loss of output from the cardiac chamber and in overfilling during diastole. The heart compensates by enlarging the capacity of the appropriate ventricle.

The left ventricle normally ejects about 70 ml. (in an adult) into the aorta during each systole and none leaks back in diastole. In severe aortic incompetence, almost half the stroke volume leaks back during diastole, so that if 70 ml. are ejected, only 40 ml. goes into the systemic circulation and 30 ml. returns to the ventricle. To compensate for this, the left ventricle enlarges so that it can eject 110 ml. during systole and, although 40 ml. may leak back, a normal output of 70 ml. per beat is regained. Normal cardiac output is achieved at the expense of considerable overwork of the left ventricle and it will inevitably fail in time unless the leaking valve is replaced.

Heart failure

Heart failure may occur suddenly when the amount of contractile muscle is reduced by occlusion of a major coronary artery or gradually when the myocardium has reached the limit of its compensatory powers. Most commonly, acute failure may be superimposed on long standing decompensation because of a final insult to a heart which has no reserves left, e.g., electrolyte imbalance, cardiac surgery or a drop in coronary blood flow consequent on an arrhythmia.

Although heart failure usually affects both the systemic and pulmonary circulations, it is helpful to consider the consequences of failure of each side of the heart separately.

Right heart failure is the common end point in patients with advanced pulmonary disease, pulmonary hypertension, mitral valve disease and atrial septal defects. The signs result from inability of the right ventricle to cope with the systemic venous return. The systemic veins become overfilled and the jugular veins become distended. The large venous sinuses in the liver share this engorgement, so that the liver becomes enlarged and palpable below the costal margin. Pressure on the bile passages may lead to jaundice. Increased pressure in the systemic veins leads to escape of fluid into the tissues and oedema occurs in dependent areas—the ankles in ambulant patients and the sacral region in patients confined to bed.

Left heart failure may be due to aortic valvular disease, systemic hypertension or coronary artery occlusion. The left ventricle is unable to pump enough blood into the aorta and blood accumulates in the pulmonary circulation. Pulmonary congestion gives rise to dyspnoea which becomes acute if pulmonary oedema should develop and the patient then coughs up pink frothy sputum. Arterial pressure may be reasonably well maintained when left heart failure is not severe but hypotension and a low pulse pressure ensue when failure becomes serious.

SYMPTOMATOLOGY

The common symptoms and signs of heart disease are discussed with reference to the alterations in haemodynamics which cause them. Many of the symptoms can occur in non-cardiac disease, but only the cardiac causes are discussed in this book. For example, haemoptysis is a common symptom of mitral stenosis but the doctor who visits a patient with haemoptysis would consider diseases of the lungs, as well as investigating disorders of the cardiovascular system.

In many heart diseases, symptoms do not appear until the compensatory mechanisms of the body have become exhausted.

For example, patients born with congenital aortic stenosis are often symptom-free during their childhood, because the left ventricle hypertrophies sufficiently to maintain an adequate output through the narrowed valve. Symptoms appear only when the left ventricle begins to fail.

In other conditions, symptoms appear in the course of disease because compensatory mechanisms do not have time to develop, e.g., coronary artery occlusion.

Some common symptoms and signs of heart disease arise from the compensatory mechanisms themselves rather than from the underlying defect. For example, in aortic stenosis, angina often develops late in the course of disease, because the muscle mass of the left ventricle has increased to a point where the available coronary blood supply is insufficient to nourish it. Symptoms and signs of heart disease due to compensatory changes which have developed as a consequence of the original defect or disease may be a warning that breakdown is imminent. When angina (p. 15) appears in the course of aortic valve disease, the patient's expectation of life is approximately 18 months.

Dyspnoea

Dyspnoea is the commonest symptom of heart disease and it is usually caused by engorgement of the pulmonary vascular bed. An increase in the amount of blood flowing into the pulmonary circulation (e.g., in septal defects and patent ductus arteriosus) or a resistance to blood flowing out of the lungs (e.g., in mitral stenosis) can alter the balance between the relative volumes of air and blood in the lungs and cause breathlessness.

Initially, dyspnoea may occur only after exercise, but as the disease progresses or the heart muscle fails, breathlessness may occur at rest. Eventually the patient is breathless even when he is lying quietly and he has to sit up to breathe comfortably. This is the stage of orthopnoea when patients are liable to attacks of pulmonary oedema (p. 14).

Cyanosis

Cyanosis is a bluish colouration of the skin and mucous membranes. It is usual to distinguish two types: central and peripheral.

Central cyanosis affects the whole body but is most easily seen in the tongue and mouth. It is produced by the mixing of a large quantity of venous blood with the systemic circulation and is most commonly seen in congenital heart defects with a right to left shunt, or with atelectasis of a portion of lung. When central cyanosis has been present for several years, clubbing of the fingers always develops for reasons which are not yet known.

Peripheral cyanosis affects the fingers and toes and sometimes the nose and ears. It is due to a low cardiac output and a sluggish peripheral circulation. As a sign of heart disease it is most commonly seen in patients whose cardiac output is reduced by some obstructive lesion, e.g., mitral stenosis, pulmonary stenosis, or constrictive pericarditis. Normally, the skin is pink because the blood flowing through it is oxygenated. When the circulation is sluggish, the tissues abstract oxygen faster than it can be supplied and the blood in the skin vessels becomes deoxygenated. This is most likely to happen in the extremities furthest from the heart—hence the name, peripheral cyanosis. It can also occur in normal people as a result of peripheral vasoconstriction in cold weather or in post-operative patients who are vaso-constricted due to hypovolaemia, pain, or a low body temperature.

The two types of cyanosis can be distinguished with certainty by measuring the oxygen content of blood from a main artery. In peripheral cyanosis, the arterial blood is normally oxygenated, whereas the oxygen content of the blood is reduced in central cyanosis.

Haemoptysis

In heart disease, haemoptysis is caused by the rupture of a small pulmonary blood vessel into the air passages. It is a common early symptom of mitral stenosis due to engorgement of the pulmonary circulation. Although the symptom is alarming to the patient, the volume of blood lost is usually small and there are no sequelae.

Haemoptysis accompanied by dyspnoea and chest pain on respiration is usually due to a pulmonary infarct. In a post-operative patient this is due to impaction of a small pulmonary embolus and, in a patient with chronic heart failure, it may be due to thrombosis in the pulmonary vascular bed.

Post-operatively, the sputum may contain old dark blood for several days if the lung was injured in the process of dividing pleural adhesions. This is often unavoidable during second operations on the thoracic cavity because adhesions have formed between the lung and chest wall after the first thoracotomy. The patient should be reassured that the sputum will become clear in a few days.

Peripheral oedema

Oedema is an excess of fluid in the tissues, of a degree sufficient to cause swelling. The site of collection of the fluid depends on gravity, and the ankles and feet swell in ambulant patients and the area over the sacrum and hips swells in bed-ridden patients.

Oedema is also a common sign of kidney or liver disease, and it may also be due to hypoproteinaemia, local injury or inflammation. In heart disease it is due to right ventricular failure. The right ventricle pumps venous blood from the body into the lungs and, when it fails, venous pressure rises and the systemic veins become engorged. Fluid seeps through the walls of venules and capillaries into the tissues and oedema appears.

Pulmonary oedema

This is a dangerous condition in which oedema fluid seeps into the alveoli, interferes with oxygen exchange and may actually 'drown' the patient. It is caused by left ventricular failure, e.g., in severe aortic stenosis. Normally the left ventricle receives blood from the pulmonary veins (via the left atrium) and pumps it into the systemic circulation. If the left ventricle fails, engorgement of the pulmonary veins and capillaries results and fluid seeps into the alveoli causing pulmonary oedema.

Pulmonary oedema can occur as an acute episode and be fatal. Following unaccustomed exertion or excitement, the patient suddenly becomes acutely breathless and coughs up copious volumes of pink frothy watery sputum. Urgent treatment is essential. The patient should be propped up, given oxygen by mask and a sedative and diuretic intravenously. This therapy will cope with a mild attack but more severe episodes may require endotracheal intubation, endobronchial suction and mechanical ventilation of the lungs with positive pressure.

Palpitations

Palpitation is an awareness of the heart beat, which is usually due to an arrhythmia. When normal rhythm changes to auricular fibrillation the patient will suddenly be conscious that his heart is racing and that its beats are irregular. Palpitation may also be caused by extra-systoles or paroxysmal tachycardia.

Angina

Angina is the name given to the severe pain produced by hypoxia of the heart muscle. It is the commonest symptom of coronary arteriosclerosis and 'angina of effort' occurs during exercise or excitement, when the heart muscle is having to do extra work but has a limited supply of oxygen-carrying blood. The pain gradually abates when the patient rests, or it can be relieved by sucking glyceryl trinitrate tablets which are believed to dilate the coronary arteries.

Angina is a crushing type of pain. Patients say they feel 'as if an iron band is being tightened round my chest', or 'as if a horse was sitting on my chest'. It often spreads into the neck and down the arms causing tingling in the fingers. Besides being the classical symptom of coronary artery occlusion or coronary insufficiency, anginal pain occurs whenever the myocardium is overworked in the presence of an inadequate coronory blood supply, e.g., as a late symptom of aortic stenosis or in fast arrhythmias.

CHAPTER 3

Cardiac Surgery

THE INVESTIGATION

Every operation on the heart is a major undertaking and the result obtained depends to a large extent on the selection of patients and on the selection of the correct procedure for each patient. Precision in diagnosis is essential and one must make a careful assessment of the state of the heart muscle, the adequacy of the pulmonary and systemic circulations, and the capacity of the lungs, liver and kidneys to cope with the extra demands imposed on them by major surgery.

Physical examination

A careful clinical examination is required to assess the patient's general appearance and physique, his colour, which may show cyanosis, the presence or absence of oedema, distension of the external jugular and other superficial veins and enlargement of the liver. The heart is palpated to assess the site and character of the apex impulse, percussed to determine cardiac size, and auscultated to detect murmurs or other abnormalities of the heart sounds. Pulse rate and rhythm and blood pressure are noted. Chest, abdomen and peripheral pulses are also examined.

Radiology

The cardiac silhouette seen in antero-posterior and oblique films of the chest gives valuable information concerning the relative size of each heart chamber (Fig. 6) and aids the diagnosis of enlargement of each. The appearance of the lungs may reveal generalised pulmonary congestion, basal congestion or pleural effusion in left heart failure, or other incidental lesions. Calcification or dilatation of the aortic arch may be revealed.

In addition, heart action is studied on a fluoroscopic screen and the excessive pulsation in the main pulmonary arteries associated with left to right shunts can be visualised.

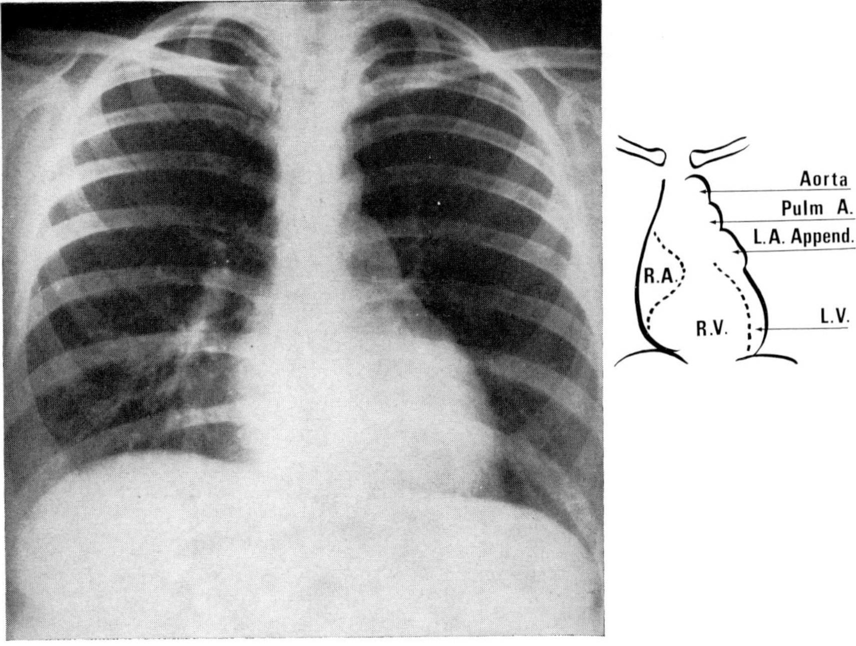

FIG. 6. The silhouette of the cardiac chambers seen on an X-ray of the thorax.

To face page 16

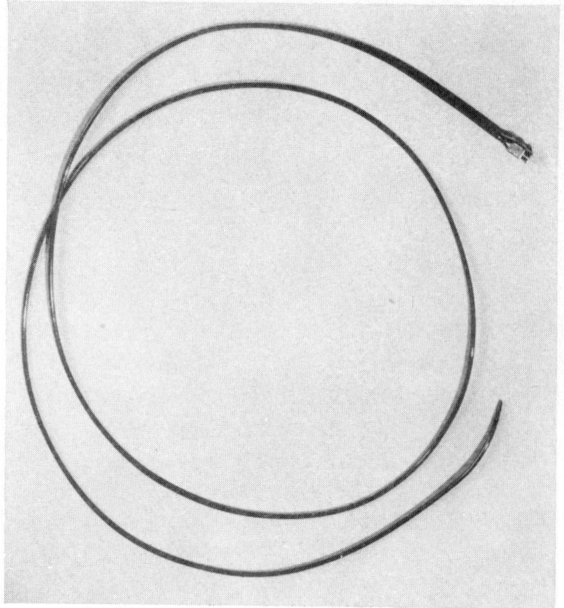

FIG. 7. A conventional cardiac catheter.

Electrocardiography

The electrocardiogram adds three items of diagnostic information. It shows the cardiac rhythm, it gives information about the size and work load of the cardiac chambers, and it can indicate to some extent whether or not the coronary circulation is adequate to meet the needs of the myocardium. Common ECG patterns are illustrated in Appendix A.

Phonocardiography

This is a record on paper of the sound waves produced by heart action and it is of value in relating the precise time of heart sounds and murmurs to the phases of the cardiac cycle.

Jugular phlebogram

This is a tracing of the pressure waves in the jugular vein. It is of some value in certain lesions affecting the right heart, but its value is limited compared with other investigations and it is now seldom used.

Cardiac catheterisation : Angiocardiography

This involves the passage of a flexible hollow radio-opaque tube (Fig. 7) along a vein into the right heart, or along an artery into the left heart. It is used for three principal purposes: (1) to measure the pressures in the cardiac chambers and great vessels, (2) to allow blood samples to be obtained from different sites in the heart and (3) to inject radio-opaque fluid so that X-rays can outline the cardiac chambers and great vessels (angiocardiography).

RIGHT HEART CATHETERISATION

On the day before this investigation, the purpose of the test should be explained to the patient, and he is given a brief outline of the procedure. He should be told that he will have to lie fairly still for about 45 minutes on an X-ray table top and that, apart from the injection of local anaesthetic, he will feel no discomfort associated with the passage of the catheter.

The patient lies on an X-ray screening table with his right arm on an arm-board. The skin over the front of the elbow is prepared with an antibacterial solution and the arm is draped with sterile sheets. The skin overlying the median antecubital vein is anaesthetised with 1 per cent lignocaine without adrenaline (i.e. 'Xylocaine Plain'). The vein is exposed through a small incision, opened between snares of fine 'Mersilene' and the cardiac catheter is introduced. A slow drip of heparinised saline (10 mg. in 500 ml. saline) is allowed to flow as soon as it is inserted. Under X-ray guidance, the radio-opaque catheter is advanced up the vein, through the right atrium and right ventricle into the main pulmonary artery. The butt end of the catheter is attached to a system of taps one of which is connected to an electromanometer for measuring pressures and another allows blood samples to be withdrawn through the catheter. The catheter is withdrawn slowly through the right heart, pausing in each chamber to take blood samples and to record pressures. The blood samples are aspirated into heparinised syringes, and the sealed syringes are immediately sent to the biochemistry laboratory for analysis of the oxygen content of the blood. In cases of congenital septal defects, the catheter can often be manipulated through the defect into the left side of the heart, thereby clearly establishing the presence, if not the size, of the septal defect.

When an angiogram is required, an angiographic catheter (which has several side holes at its tip instead of a single end hole) is substituted for the conventional catheter. A pressurised injector loaded with radio-opaque fluid (1 ml. per kg. body weight) is connected to the catheter and a bolus is injected into the heart. A record of the passage of this fluid through the heart and pulmonary vessels is made on ciné-X-ray film (i.e., a ciné-angiogram). The angioatheter is removed, the vein is ligated, and the skin wound is closed with one or two interrupted sutures.

Cardiac catheterisation is conducted with full sterile precautions as in an operating theatre, and an antibiotic (ampicillin) is given to minimise the risk of bacterial endocarditis. The first dose of 500 mg. is administered 2 to 3 hours before catheterisation and subsequent doses of 250 mg. are given 6-hourly for 36 hours.

LEFT HEART CATHETERISATION

This is a slightly more hazardous procedure than right heart catheterisation because it requires the introduction of a catheter into an artery and, during angiography, the contrast medium may reach the coronary and cerebral circulations in relatively high concentrations. The patient experiences a general sensation of warmth, and is sometimes sick, and many physicians prefer to perform left heart angiography under general anaesthesia. Patients undergoing left heart catheterisation should be prepared for a general anaesthetic in case this is necessary.

There are two methods commonly used to introduce a catheter into an artery.

Percutaneous catheterisation (Seldinger technique, Figure 8). The

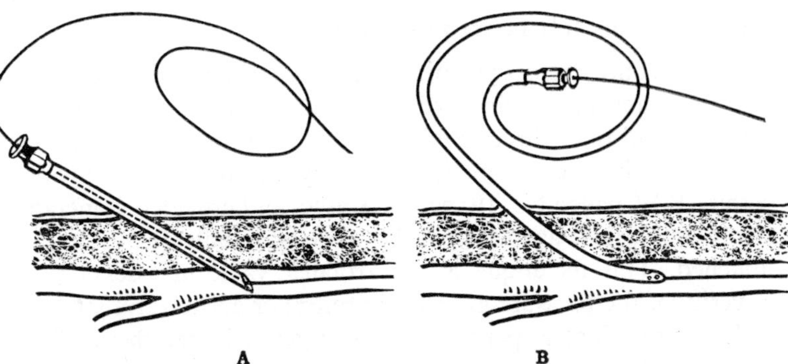

FIG. 8. Percutaneous catheterisation. A Introduction of the needle and guide wire. B Introduction of the catheter along the guide wire.

skin over the femoral artery or, in some cases (e.g., coarctation) the brachial artery, is anaesthetised with 1 per cent plain lignocaine, and the skin is punctured with a pointed scalpel. A thin-walled wide bore needle is introduced into the artery so that it points towards the heart. When the needle is situated in the lumen of the artery as shown by jets of blood coming from its butt, a fine flexible 'guide' wire is introduced through the needle and pushed a few inches up the artery. The needle is then withdrawn leaving the 'guide' wire in the artery. A radio-opaque flexible catheter with a tapered tip is threaded over the 'guide' wire and pushed through the cut in the skin into the artery and the wire can then be removed and the catheter manipulated towards the heart. The butt end of the catheter is connected to pressure measuring equipment and a source of heparin-saline for flushing and sampling syringes. A skilled operator can usually direct the catheter tip through the aortic valve into the left ventricle where pressures and samples are obtained and angiography can be done. When the procedure is finished, the catheter is withdrawn and firm pressure is maintained over the site of the arterial puncture for several minutes to prevent haematoma formation.

Open Arteriotomy. In very fat patients or in children, percutaneous catheterisation may be difficult and it is often better to expose the artery through a small incision and the catheter is introduced through a small cut in the vessel. When the catheter has been withdrawn, this arteriotomy must be carefully repaired using 5/O or 6/O non-absorbable sutures.

Percutaneous left heart puncture

When the only haemodynamic information required is a record of the pressures in certain cardiac chambers or great vessels, the simplest and most direct method is to introduce a needle directly into these chambers. This is a perfectly safe procedure provided a thin (B.W. gauge No. 19) needle is used, and provided vulnerable areas such as the atrio-ventricular node or bundle of His are not touched. This technique is of particular value in assessing the severity of the pressure gradient in mitral or aortic valve stenosis.

The procedure is performed under general anaesthesia. With the patient on his back and his head extended and turned to one side, a long (20 cm.) needle is entered through the skin of the

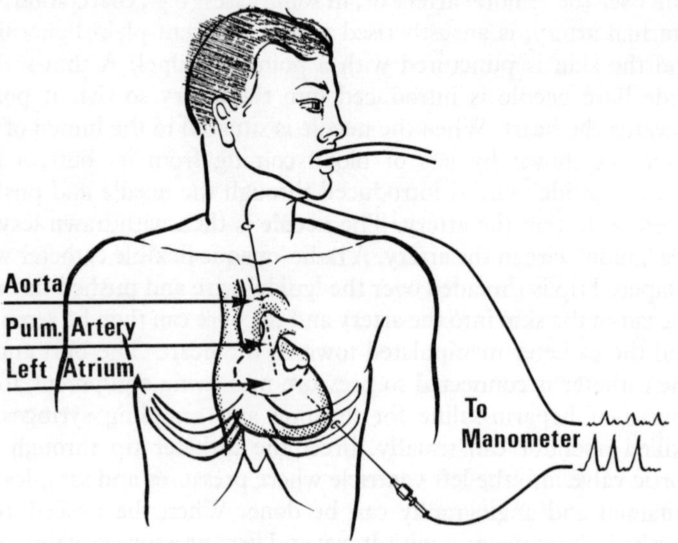

FIG. 9. Percutaneous needle puncture of the left ventricle, left atrium and great vessels.

supra-sternal notch and advanced downwards towards the heart in a direction parallel to the trachea. The needle penetrates in turn the arch of the aorta, the main pulmonary artery and, finally, the left atrium. A second needle is inserted through the skin where the apex beat is felt and is passed through the intercostal space into the left ventricle (Fig. 9). Pressures and blood samples are taken from the left ventricle, left atrium, pulmonary artery and aorta, then the needles are withdrawn.

Nursing care after cardiac catheterisation or left heart puncture

Most patients are not upset by cardiac catheterisation and require no special care afterwards. However, ill patients and those who have had a general anaesthetic are liable to develop dangerous arrhythmias and hypotension.

Three groups of patients are liable to develop cardio-vascular instability after catheterisation: (1) those with severe pulmonary hypertension, (2) those with advanced rheumatic valvular disease affecting more than one valve and (3) those with cyanotic congenital heart disease. These patients should be nursed in an intensive care area for a few hours during which time the ECG is monitored and pulse rate and blood pressure are charted quarter hourly until the vital functions have stabilised.

An X-ray of chest should be taken after left heart puncture, to exclude the presence of pneumothorax or haemopericardium.

Preparation for Surgery

The successful outcome of major surgical procedures depends to a certain extent on careful pre-operative preparation of the patient.

If the patient has developed heart failure, a period of rest and medical treatment (digoxin and diuretics) is necessary. Anaemia must be corrected and the function of the liver, lungs and kidneys must be assessed by special tests. Bad teeth should be extracted or filled under antibiotic cover, the patient should be taught deep breathing exercises, and the importance of correct breathing after operation should be explained.

Nurses and doctors sometimes overlook the fact that a surgical operation is a unique and often a frightening experience to the patient. The psychological preparation of the patient is an important part of pre-operative care. This is particularly important when the patient will require post-operative care in an intensive therapy area. The patient should be shown where he will wake up and should be allowed to try on an oxygen mask. The various monitoring attachments are explained to him (e.g. ECG wires, rectal temperature probes, etc.). If mechanical ventilation is going to be used post-operatively, this should be explained beforehand, as well as the purpose of chest drainage tubes and the bladder catheter. A tranquilliser drug during the day and a sedative at night is often required for a few days before operation.

Scope and Techniques of Cardiac Surgery

The three types of heart disease which account for the major part of the cardiac surgeon's work load are (1) chronic rheumatic disease of the heart valves, (2) congenital defects and (3) occlusive disease of the coronary arteries.

Lesions of the great vessels such as coarctation of the aorta and aneurysms of the aortic arch also come within the province of the cardio-vascular surgeon, because the techniques involved are similar to those used in operating upon the heart. Tumours of the heart are rare and occur in one patient in every 500 seen at a cardiac surgical clinic. They are usually benign and can be excised quite easily. Wounds of the heart are equally rare in civilian practice. In most cases the principal danger is cardiac tamponade (p. 85), but treatment presents no difficulties, provided tamponade is recognised in time. Constrictive pericarditis and the rare pericardial cysts also come within the scope of cardiac surgery.

Techniques in cardiac surgery

Operations on the heart can be undertaken while the heart is still beating, closed heart surgery, or while the circulation to the brain and the rest of the body is maintained by heart-lung bypass techniques, open heart surgery. The choice of method depends on the nature of the lesion and on the amount of operating time required.

CLOSED-HEART SURGERY

The commonest type of operation performed in closed heart surgery is mitral valvotomy. In cases of mitral stenosis, the surgeon introduces his finger and special instruments into the beating heart and, working by touch, divides the adhesions which have produced narrowing of the mitral valve.

Certain operations designed to improve the blood supply to the heart muscle in patients with coronary artery disease also come into this category, e.g., Vineberg's operation (p. 66), as do some operations on the great vessels, e.g., correction of coarctation and closure of a patent ductus arteriosus.

OPEN-HEART SURGERY (HEART-LUNG BYPASS)

Open-heart surgery necessitates the use of a heart-lung machine to maintain the patient's circulation while the heart is being repaired. This gives the exposure and operating time required for repair of intracardiac congenital defects and valve replacement operations which are performed under direct vision with one or more chambers of the heart opened.

Heart-lung machines take over the functions of the heart and lungs for a period varying from 15 minutes to 3 hours or more depending on the complexity of the intracardiac procedure. The machine oxygenates the blood and pumps it through the systemic circulation. The patient is heparinised before connection is made to the heart-lung machine, so that blood will not clot in the extra-corporeal circuit.

The circuit of a heart-lung machine is made up as follows (Fig.

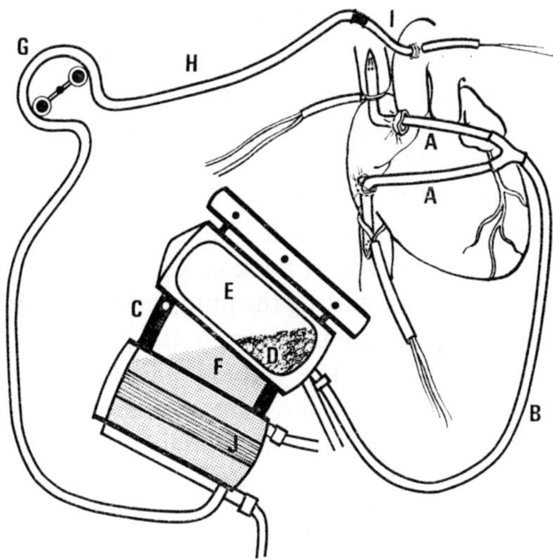

FIG. 10. The circuit for heart-lung bypass (see text, page 24).

10). Two caval cannulae (A) are introduced into the superior and inferior venae cavae to collect the venous blood on its way to the heart and divert it through the venous line (B) to the oxygenator (C). This lies about 18 in. below the patient so that the venous blood runs into it by gravity-siphonage. There are several types of oxygenator, but the most widely used is a specially designed plastic bag divided into three compartments. Venous blood passes into the first compartment (D) where oxygen is bubbled into the blood to oxygenate it. The second compartment (E) is filled with a fine mesh of steel wool or nylon, coated with a silicone anti-foam preparation so that the bubbles will burst and the oxygenated blood will leave this compartment free from bubbles. The third compartment (F) is a reservoir to collect the blood and the pump (G) forces it along the tubing (H) to the arterial cannula (I). The pump consists of electrically driven rollers which compress the tubing leading from the reservoir (F) to the patient, and the blood is forcibly 'milked' through the tubing of the arterial line into the systemic arterial circulation. The pumping rate can be varied so as to maintain a normal blood pressure in the patient's arteries. The arterial blood is usually returned to the ascending aorta through an arterial cannula introduced through a purse string suture (I). At some point in the circuit, blood passes through a heat exchanger (J) so that its temperature can be controlled.

Before use, the circuit is 'primed' (i.e. filled) with Ringer's solution (or 5 per cent dextrose-water). The consequent dilution of the patient's blood does no harm and the extra fluid is excreted by the kidney in the early post-operative period. In children and small adults, the amount of fluid necessary to fill the circuit (2·5 to 3·0 litres) could cause too much haemodilution and one or two units of donor blood are included in these cases.

Bypass is instituted by starting the pump and releasing the clamp on the venous line. The venous return to the heart flows out to the oxygenator, the heart quickly empties and the patient's blood pressure and arterial blood flow are maintained by the blood pumped back into the aorta. Tapes are tightened around the caval cannulae soon after bypass is instituted.

The aortic arterial pressure closes the aortic valve, and the heart remains empty except for some blood which passes through the coronary circulation to the right atrium via the coronary sinus. This blood is aspirated by a special sucker (the cardiotomy sucker) when the heart is opened and returned to the circuit through a side-opening in the oxygenator. Coronary perfusion is therefore maintained by the pump while the heart is being operated on. However, operations on the aortic valve involve placing a clamp on the ascending aorta just proximal to the arterial cannula (Fig. 11)

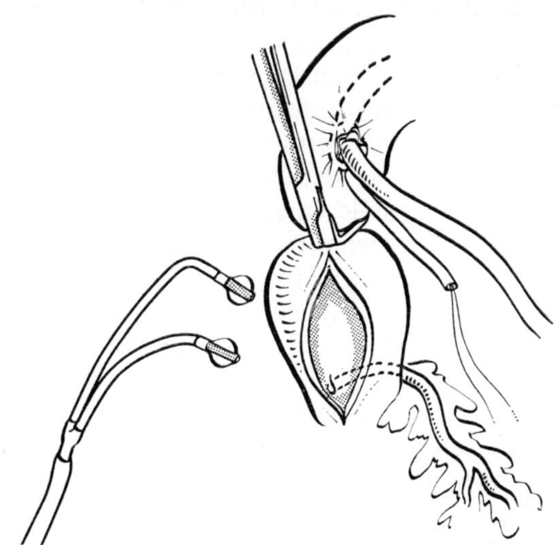

FIG. 11. The aortic incision for aortic valve surgery and for access to the orifices of the coronary arteries. The cannulae used for perfusion of the coronary arteries are shown on the left.

and this cuts off the coronary arteries from the supply of oxygenated blood. Separate provision for maintenance of the coronary circulation is made by inserting small cannulae into the orifices of the two coronary arteries as soon as the aorta is opened and a side branch of the main arterial line conveys blood to perfuse the myocardium.

In some operations, it is not necessary or desirable to maintain coronary perfusion continuously. If coronary blood flow is stopped, the heart slows down and stops beating completely after about 10 minutes. In this inactive condition, it requires very little oxygen and, provided it does not have to work, the heart muscle will tolerate cessation of coronary blood flow for up to 60 minutes. This state of anoxic cardiac arrest offers nearly ideal conditions for operations within the heart, i.e. the heart is relaxed, flaccid, and almost bloodless. It is therefore common practice to cross-clamp the ascending aorta for 30 to 40 minutes in the course of many open-heart operations but coronary perfusion is essential during long operations in order to prevent myocardial damage.

Hypothermia

If the temperature of the body is artificially lowered, its metabolic rate falls and the tissues require less oxygen and consequently less blood flow. Hibernating animals use this principle to survive the winter without eating, and cardiac surgeons use hypothermia without heart-lung bypass for short open heart operations such as the repair of small atrial septal defects.

The technique is as follows: after the patient has been anaesthetised he is cooled to a temperature of 30°C by immersion in ice-water or by blowing cold air over him. The heart is exposed, the venae cavae are taped or clamped to stop venous return, the aorta is cross-clamped and the heart is opened. At 30°C the circulation can be arrested for only eight minutes because a longer period causes damage to the brain and kidneys.

Hypothermia can also be used with heart-lung bypass for long operations. The temperature of the blood is regulated as it passes through the heart-lung machine, and the lower pumping rate which is sufficient to maintain the patient's circulation reduces the rate of damage to blood corpuscles pumped round and round the artificial circuit.

Prostheses used in cardiac surgery

The striking developments in plastics and man-made fibres which have occurred during the past 20 years, have been applied in the manufacture of artificial heart valves and in making patches used in the repair of large septal defects.

Material implanted in a patient must be biologically inert, i.e., it should not interact either physically or chemically with the body tissues and fluids. If it did so, it would provoke a sterile inflammatory response and fail to be incorporated in the body tissues. The two commonly used fabrics which have this property are Teflon and Dacron (which is the American name for Terylene).

These fabrics form a scaffold or framework in the body into which the surrounding tissues can grow. When a Dacron patch is sewn in to close a septal defect, thrombus forms on each surface and in the weave of the material and cannot peel off as an embolus.

During the next six months fibroblasts replace the thrombus with fibrous tissue and the cloth becomes completely covered by a smooth lining similar to the endocardium.

The same process of incorporation occurs with modern artificial valves. The older types of artificial valves had bare metal exposed, and the thrombus which formed on the polished metal surface could separate and produce an embolus. Cloth-covered valves are now preferred because of the very low incidence of embolism which follows their use.

The artificial valves in common use (Fig. 12) bear little resemblance to the valves they replace but attempts to manufacture more natural valves have failed because the repeated flexion or hingeing action causes them to break up. It seems likely, however, that further advances in technology will develop materials capable of standing up to normal stresses and 'leaflet' valves will then become available.

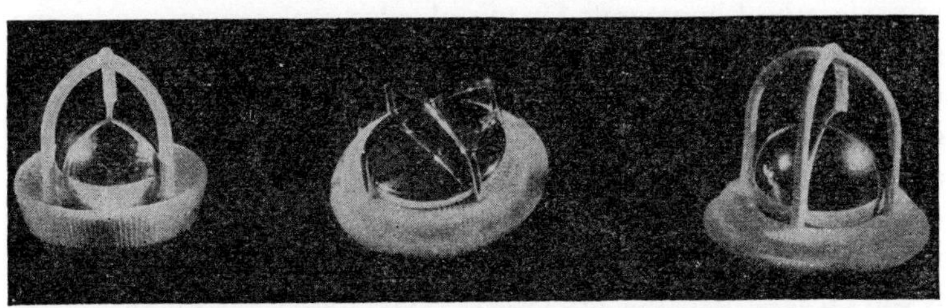

FIG. 12. Starr-Edwards prosthetic valves for replacement of the aortic, tricuspid and mitral valves (from left to right).

Suture materials

These are now as varied and as sophisticated as the prostheses which they hold in place and there are too many varieties to refer to them in detail. The important point is that prostheses must be fixed in place by unabsorbable sutures and, while many surgeons still prefer silk for this purpose, most use the newer materials such as Terylene (Mersilene) or plastic coated sutures (Tefdek, Tycron, etc.).

Homograft valves

Although a valve replacement operation may save a patient who would otherwise have died, mechanical valves still fall short of the ideal substitute in two important respects. First we do not know how long they will last, and reports of malfunction in some of the earlier prostheses have already been published. Secondly, thrombus embolism remains a hazard to patients with an artificial valve, and anticoagulant therapy must be continued indefinitely.

For these reasons, some surgeons prefer to use preserved homograft valves (taken from cadavers) for valve replacement surgery. Anticoagulants are not necessary after operation where a homograft valve has been used, and the results of aortic valve replacement with homografts have been excellent in the few centres where this technique has been perfected. It has not yet proved possible to use a mitral homograft for mitral valve replacement, and some surgeons use an aortic homograft fixed to a plastic frame and sewn into the mitral annulus. Others have used autogenous fascia lata on a similar frame and, although the results of these procedures are still under evaluation, the early reports are encouraging.

However, shrinkage and calcification have been found to occur in homograft valves and long term results must be awaited before it can be said that they are clearly preferable to prosthetic valves.

Transplantation of the heart

Cardiac surgery took a dramatic leap forward in 1967 when Professor Christian Barnard successfully transplanted a human heart. The bold application of established organ transplantation techniques to heart surgery has introduced new possibilities in the treatment of incurable heart disease.

Immuno-suppressive methods are still imperfect and routine cardiac transplantation is not yet possible. However, transplantation of the heart is now technically feasible and it seems probable that the problem of rejection will be solved during the next decade.

At the present time, a heart transplant is the only method of cure for three groups of patients: (1) children born with complex congenital cardiac defects, (2) patients with multivalvular rheumatic heart disease in whom the myocardium has irrecoverably exhausted its compensatory powers and (3) cases of extensive coronary occlusive disease where the myocardium is being progressively replaced by fibrous tissue.

Transplantation of the heart is performed as follows. The chest is opened through a median sternotomy incision and the pericardium is opened widely. The venae cavae and aorta are cannulated and the patient is put on conventional heart-lung bypass. The aorta and pulmonary artery are clamped 5 cm. above the heart which is then excised so as to leave in situ the posterior parts of both atria, which receive the venae cavae and the pulmonary veins. As little as possible of the patient's atria is left, because they are deprived of a coronary blood supply, but the sino-atrial node is retained.

At the same time, the donor's heart is removed by a second surgical team and the posterior walls of both atria are excised together with the major veins. The donor heart is sutured in place, starting with the inter-atrial septum, sewing donor atrium to recipient atrium, and finally the aorta and pulmonary arteries are sutured end to end.

The healthy heart can tolerate interruption of its coronary blood supply for one hour, so the aortic anastomosis must be completed within this time and the clamp on the patient's aorta is then released to allow coronary perfusion of the donor heart.

Immuno-suppressive therapy is started some time before operation, if possible. Most surgeons use a combination of steroids, Azathioprine and anti-lymphocytic serum or globulin. The initial high dosage of these agents is reduced during the next 10 days, but it is increased again if any evidence of rejection appears.

The results of transplantation of the heart, at present, must limit its application to a very carefully selected group of patients for whom no alternative therapy is available. Its wider application will follow further elucidation of the problems related to homograft rejection.

CHAPTER 4

Rheumatic Heart Disease

Rheumatic carditis is a serious complication of acute rheumatic fever and damage to the mitral, aortic or tricuspid valves may result. A slow progressive fibrosis leads to increasing malfunction and mitral valve lesions caused by rheumatic fever constitute the largest group of cases requiring cardiac surgery. At the present time, about 300 operations per week are performed for rheumatic valvular disease in Britain, and, although rheumatic fever is much less common today than it was 20 years ago, a further 20 years will probably pass before rheumatic valvular disease becomes uncommon.

The natural history of the disease

Rheumatic heart disease is an abnormal tissue reaction to the toxins of a haemolytic streptococcal infection. The classical acute illness is characterised by a high temperature and joint pains, and it occurs as a sequel to a streptococcal sore throat. Children and adolescents are principally affected and rheumatic fever is rare in infants and uncommon in adults. About two-thirds of those who have rheumatic fever in childhood develop permanent valve damage, and in two-thirds of these it is severe enough to warrant surgery.

At the time of the acute illness the leaflets of the valves become inflamed and swollen and may partially stick together, and the chordae tendineae become swollen and thickened.

This initial damage to the valve leaflets is followed by a very slow process of fibrosis and scarring which relentlessly distorts the valve leaflets and 10 years or more usually elapses before the symptoms and signs of valve damage appear. Because the valvular changes are slow to develop and because the heart muscle can compensate by hypertrophying for many years, symptoms do not usually become severe until the patients are in their thirties. Eventually, the myocardium can no longer compensate for the narrowed or leaky valve and symptoms of cardiac failure appear.

The mitral and aortic valves are the ones most commonly damaged by rheumatic fever. Tricuspid valve disease is much less common, and the pulmonary valve is very rarely affected.

Mitral Valve Disease

Mitral stenosis. This is the commonest form of rheumatic valvular disease. The narrowed valve impedes blood flow from left atrium to left ventricle and blood accumulates in the pulmonary circulation. The left atrium enlarges to try and force blood through the narrow valve opening but this is relatively ineffective and the right ventricle has to supply the force necessary to push blood through the mitral valve, having first pumped it through the lungs (Fig. 4). The right ventricle therefore becomes hypertrophied and the pulmonary circulation is constantly overfilled with blood.

Mitral incompetence. In this condition the valve does not close properly and blood leaks back into the left atrium with each contraction of the left ventricle. This produces the same effects in the pulmonary circulation and right ventricle as mitral stenosis, but, in addition, the left ventricle enlarges and hypertrophies to compensate for the leak of blood through the incompetent valve. Under normal conditions, the left ventricle pumps about 70 ml. of blood into the aorta with each contraction. If 30 ml. squirt back into the left atrium through an incompetent valve, the ventricle will have to pump 100 ml. with each systole in order to maintain normal aortic flow. It therefore enlarges to accommodate this volume and the myocardium becomes hypertrophied. At the same time, the left atrium stretches to accommodate the leak-back.

Mitral stenosis and incompetence frequently occur together but whether there is stenosis, incompetence, or both, the pulmonary circulation is constantly overfilled, and progressive changes take place in the pulmonary blood vessels. The initial change is a thickening of the walls of the small vessels and, as this process continues, the vessels become narrowed and offer increased resistance to blood flow. The right ventricle undergoes progressive hypertrophy and, over the years, blood pressure rises in the pulmonary artery and pulmonary hypertension results.

Symptoms and signs

Dyspnoea. As the valvular disease progresses, the patient experiences breathlessness on exertion which grows gradually more severe as the years pass. Breathlessness is sometimes precipitated by pregnancy because, during the last four months of pregnancy, the heart has to pump 25 per cent more blood than normal and the obstruction produced by the narrowed valve becomes more significant.

Fatigue. The stenosed valve limits cardiac output and patients tire easily, e.g., housewives are progressively less able to manage their chores and become very tired by nightfall.

Haemoptysis. This is common in the early stages of the disease but less common in the late stages because the pulmonary vessels become thicker walled and less likely to bleed.

Palpitations. This is a fluttering sensation in the chest which makes the patient aware of the heart beat. It occurs when the beat is irregular and by far the commonest cause is auricular fibrillation which occurs in 40 per cent of all cases of mitral valve disease. In this condition, the all-in-one contraction of the atrium which normally occurs with each heart beat is replaced by irregular contractions of different areas of atrial muscle which contract independently and without any concerted rhythm.

Systemic embolism. In mitral valve disease, blood is held up in the left atrium and it may clot on the wall of this chamber. A portion of this thrombus can break loose and it is then pumped out into the aorta as an embolus. This embolus is swept along by the blood stream until it blocks an artery of similar size and the blood supply to the organ supplied by that artery is abruptly cut off (Chap. 22).

Surgical treatment

Before cardiac surgery was possible, these patients developed progressive cardiac failure which eventually ended in death from congestive heart failure. It is now possible to perform an operation which can offer the patient many more years of happy and comfortable life.

The operations available are mitral valvotomy, mitral valvuloplasty and mitral valve replacement. The choice of operation depends on the state of the valve. For pure mitral stenosis, closed mitral valvotomy is the treatment of choice. If the valve is incompetent it must usually be replaced by an artificial valve. In a very few cases it is possible to repair the valve by cutting adhesions between the leaflets or by taking a tuck in a leaking valve (i.e., valvuloplasty). If the valve is both stenosed and incompetent, replacement with an artificial valve is necessary.

There are no absolute contra-indications to operation apart from serious concurrent disease, but major cardiac surgery should only be undertaken in patients whose symptoms are significant, or in whom diagnostic tests show that progressive heart failure is imminent. If operation is delayed too long, the operative risk increases and the post-operative management becomes more difficult—in other words, the best results are obtained when operation is undertaken timeously.

MITRAL VALVOTOMY

This is a simple operation performed for mitral stenosis in which the valve is 'split' blindly with instruments while the heart is still beating, i.e., it is a 'closed-heart' operation. It is a short operation ($1\frac{1}{2}$ hours) which is not usually followed by any major cardiovascular or pulmonary complications and no special pre-operative preparations are necessary.

Technique. The heart is approached through the left side of the chest, using either an antero-lateral or a lateral incision through the fifth intercostal space (Fig. 13). The left lung is retracted back-

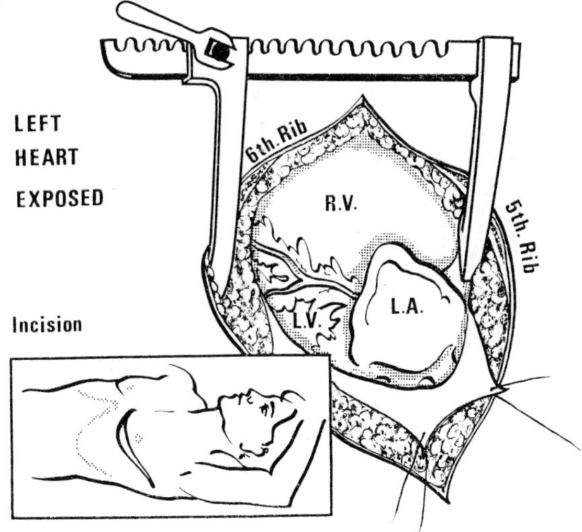

FIG. 13. Exposure of the left side of the heart for closed-heart mitral valvotomy.

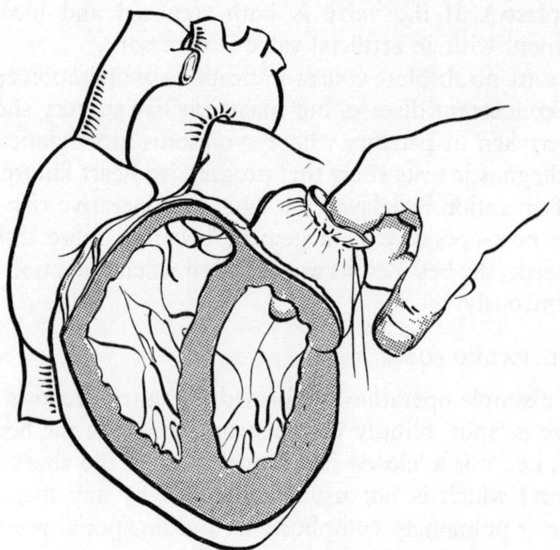

FIG. 14. Mitral valvotomy: splitting the fused mitral leaflets with the finger tip.

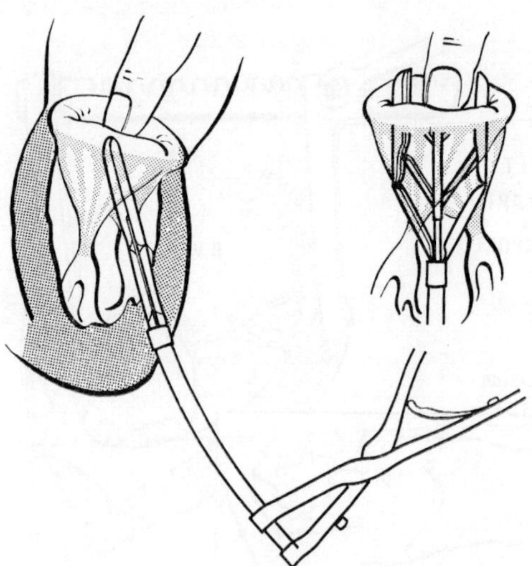

FIG. 15. Mitral valvotomy: instrumental relief of a stenosed mitral valve using Tubb's valve dilator.

wards and the pericardial sac is opened in front of the phrenic nerve, from the apex of the heart to the main pulmonary artery. This exposes the side of the left atrium, the atrial appendage, and the left ventricle. The left atrial appendage is an extension of the main cavity of the left atrium and it is usually possible to apply a clamp or purse-string suture across the region where it joins the left atrium proper, so that an opening can be cut into it large enough to admit the index finger. When the finger is introduced, the clamp is released and the finger acts as a plug to stop blood loss (Fig. 14). The orifice of the stenosed valve feels like a button-hole—a slit of about 1 cm. in length, the normal valve opening being about 3 to 4 cm. in diameter. Firm pressure with the finger will sometimes tear the adhesions between the valve leaflets and recreate an adequate orifice. In most cases this is not possible and it is necessary to use an instrument to separate the leaflets. A Tubb's dilator is used and Figure 15 shows how it is introduced into the heart through a small incision at the apex of the left ventricle. When its tip is in the mitral orifice, the dilator is opened and the valve is split. Thereafter, the instrument and finger are removed and the heart is sewn up using 2/O Mersilene.

Standing post-operative orders. Immediately on return from theatre, a team of nurses should do the following (Fig. 16).

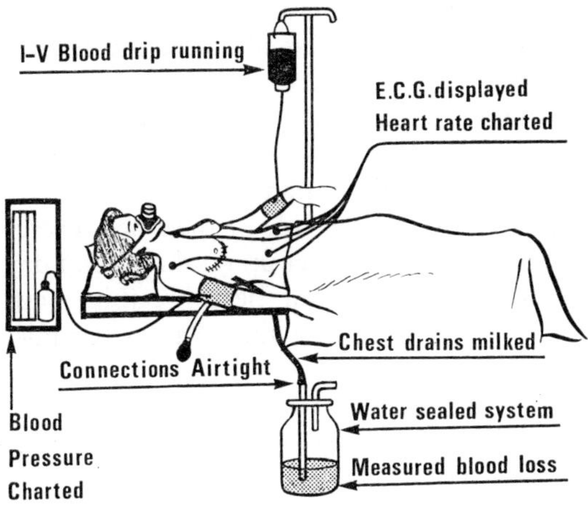

FIG. 16. The drawing emphasises the important points in post-operative management after mitral valvotomy.

1. Lay the patient flat, ensure that the airway is clear and that respiratory movements are free.
2. Measure and record the blood pressure and heart rate.
3. Give oxygen, by Edinburgh mask (4 litres/min.).
4. Ensure that the blood drip is running.
5. Milk the chest drains and chart the blood loss every 15 minutes.

It is usual to chart TPR, BP, apex rate and blood loss quarter-hourly for about 24 hours, then 4-hourly thereafter.

The patient's chest should be X-rayed to confirm re-expansion of the left lung.

The patient can usually be propped up two to four hours after leaving theatre, provided the blood pressure is adequate, i.e., above 110 mm.

Sips of water can be given (up to 60 ml./hr) as soon as the patient is fully awake. Deep breathing and coughing should be encouraged and the medical team will prescribe appropriate analgesia to relieve pain. Analgesic drugs are usually given in small frequent doses intravenously, e.g., 2 to 4 mg. morphine sulphate or 5 to 10 mg. pethidine hydrochloride every hour at first.

Blood replacement is continued until it is evident that intra-thoracic bleeding has stopped. This is usually about six hours after theatre, but the intravenous drip should be continued with 500 ml. of 5 per cent dextrose-water for a further 8 to 12 hours. The volume of blood replaced should exceed the measured loss by about 20 per cent.

Oxygen therapy can usually be discontinued after four hours, although older patients, or those with pulmonary hypertension, may require more prolonged administration.

Most patients can sit on the side of their bed, exercising their legs, by the next day and may get up on the second day.

The importance of encouraging deep breathing and coughing during the first few days after thoracotomy cannot be over-emphasised.

The two chief hazards of this operation are (1) embolism, (2) production of mitral incompetence. About 15 per cent of cases have thrombus in the left atrium and embolism may occur if this is dislodged into the left ventricle. Mitral incompetence will be produced if the valve splits in the wrong place, i.e., a leaflet gets torn. If this should occur and the incompetence is serious, replacement of the damaged valve with an artificial valve will become necessary.

Re-stenosis. It has been found that in about 20 per cent of patients who had a mitral valvotomy more than 10 years ago, symptoms have reappeared because the valve has re-stenosed. A second valvotomy may be possible but many of these patients ultimately require valve replacement.

MITRAL VALVE REPLACEMENT

This is the operation of choice for mitral incompetence or for those cases of mitral stenosis in whom the valve is badly scarred or calcified. Heart-lung bypass is required because operation is performed with the left atrium opened. This is a more major undertaking than closed mitral valvotomy and it carries a greater mortality and morbidity risk.

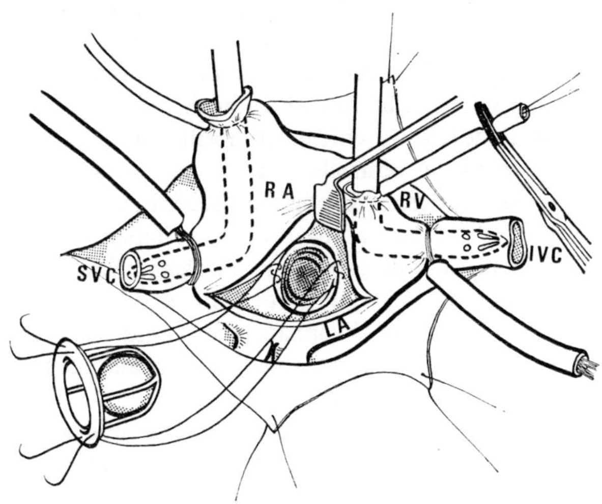

FIG. 17. Mitral valve replacement: the patient is on heart-lung bypass; the left atrium has been opened from the right side just in front of the right pulmonary veins.

Technique. The usual incision is a median sternotomy, and, while the chest is being opened, another member of the surgical team inserts a cannula into the radial artery to monitor arterial blood pressure, and a second cannula into the inferior vena cava (via the saphenous vein at the groin) to monitor the central venous pressure. At the same time the heart-lung machine is prepared and 'primed' with Ringer-lactate solution.

When the heart has been exposed, the patient is heparinised, cannulae are placed in the venae cavae via the right atrium and in the ascending aorta through a purse-string suture. The cannulae are connected to the arterial and venous connections from the heart-lung machine and bypass is commenced. With the patient's circulation taken over by the extra-corporeal circuit, the aorta is cross-clamped just above the coronary arteries and the left atrium is opened widely (Fig. 17). The mitral valve is inspected and a plastic repair of the leaflets is performed if this seems possible. Usually, however, the deformed valve is excised and the appropriate size of artificial valve sewn in place with 2/O Mersilene sutures. The left atriotomy is then closed and the heart is allowed to fill with blood by releasing the tapes around the venae cavae. Great care is taken to remove all the air from the heart by using wide bore needles placed at the root of the aorta and at the apex of the left ventricle. The aortic clamp is then released and coronary blood flow is restored. The heart may begin to contract again but more usually it develops ventricular fibrillation. A defibrillating shock is applied to the ventricles, and, when the heart is beating strongly, bypass is progressively discontinued. Finally, the cannulae are removed from the cavae and aorta and the heparin is neutralised by an intravenous dose of protamine sulphate. The pericardium is only partially closed to avoid risk of tamponade and the sternum is re-approximated with steel wire and the wound is closed. Drainage tubes are led from the anterior mediastinum and the pericardial cavity to a water-sealed collection system.

Post-operative complications. Apart from the complications which can occur in any patient undergoing thoracotomy and bypass surgery (viz. haemorrhage, pulmonary atelectasis, wound and pulmonary infection), cases of mitral valve replacement require careful supervision of their fluid and electrolyte balance. Many have been on maintenance diuretic therapy which tends to cause potassium depletion. Transient arrhythmias are common and call for careful monitoring of the ECG and treatment with digitalis or anti-arrhythmic drugs as required. The cardiac output tends to be low during the first few days after mitral valve replacement, and in some cases myocardial 'stimulant' drugs such as isoprenaline

('Suscardia') are required as a slow intravenous drip for 24 to 48 hours, (2·0 mg. in 500 ml. at 5 to 10 drops/min.).

Aortic Valve Disease

The aortic valve is less commonly affected by rheumatic fever than the mitral, but once symptoms have appeared, deterioration is more rapid and the expectation of life is shorter. This is because stenosis or incompetence of the aortic valve overloads the main pumping chamber of the heart, the left ventricle.

The haemodynamic effects of aortic stenosis and incompetence have already been described in Chapter 4. Stenosis causes concentric hypertrophy of the left ventricle with very little increase in its external size until heart failure appears. Aortic incompetence, on the other hand, leads to the development of a greatly enlarged left ventricle which shows an increase in both muscle mass and overall size.

With both stenosis and incompetence, the occurrence of episodes of pulmonary oedema indicates left ventricular failure, and operation must not be delayed.

Symptoms and signs

Dyspnoea on effort is the commonest symptom. Black-outs or syncopal attacks can occur on exertion or after bending down and these are caused by a reduction in cardiac output which produces relative cerebral ischaemia. Syncopal attacks occurring late in the course of the disease may signify an episode of ventricular tachycardia which is an ominous sign. Acute pulmonary oedema occurs when the left ventricle fails.

Angina pectoris is also a late symptom. The low cardiac output which occurs in these patients gives a poor coronary flow which is insufficient to meet the demands of the hypertrophied left ventricle and the relative myocardial ischaemia gives rise to anginal pain.

A provisional diagnosis can be made from the signs of an enlarged left ventricle with a harsh systolic murmur at the aortic valve area. Diagnosis is confirmed by left heart catheterisation which demonstrates the pressure gradient between the aorta and left ventricle during systole and by angiography which outlines the narrowed valve.

Surgical treatment

Blind valvotomy has no place in the treatment of aortic valve disease because the risk of producing incompetence is high, re-stenosis would occur within a few years, and adequate relief of stenosis could not be achieved with certainty.

The standard treatment of aortic stenosis and/or incompetence is replacement by an artificial valve or homograft.

Technique. Operation is performed through a median sternotomy. The pericardium is incised vertically from the diaphragm to the remnants of the thymus, and venae cavae and aorta are cannulated for heart-lung bypass.

With the circulation maintained by the heart-lung machine, the aorta is cross-clamped just proximal to the arterial cannula. A suction cannula is placed in the left ventricle through a small incision at the apex, and the ascending aorta is opened with an oblique incision four centimetres in length. The diseased valve is excised and sutures are placed in the aortic annulus to secure the artificial valve (Fig. 18). 18-20 double armed sutures of 2/0 Mersilene are placed in both the annulus and the prosthesis before the latter is slid down into place below the orifices of the coronary arteries. The aortic incision is then closed with a continuous stitch of 3/0 Mersilene.

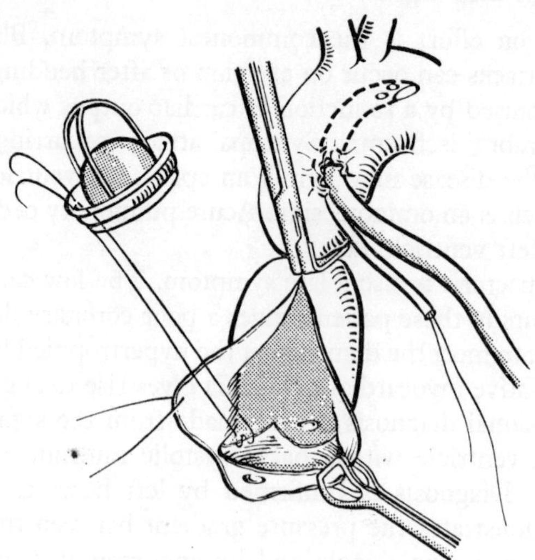

FIG. 18. Aortic valve replacement.

The heart and root of the aorta are allowed to fill with blood and trapped air is vented through a wide-bore needle in the aortic incision and through the left ventricular cannula. When it is certain that all the air has been evacuated, the aortic clamp is released. This restores coronary blood flow and, after a few minutes, the flaccid heart regains tone and fibrillates. A defibrillator shock is applied to restore ventricular contraction. Rarely, the heart will beat spontaneously without requiring electrical defibrillation.

In the light of our present experience, the maximum safe period of arrest of the coronary circulation is one hour. Patients who are over 40 years of age or who have coronary artery disease can sustain myocardial damage with even shorter periods of arrest and cannulae for perfusion of the coronary arteries are prepared before the aorta is cross-clamped. If the surgeon finds that the operating time on the valve will exceed 30 or 40 minutes, the coronary arteries are cannulated and perfused.

In older patients and in those who showed evidence of incipient cardiac failure before operation, the heart may be slow to take over the circulation from the heart-lung machine at the end of the intra-cardiac part of the operation. In these cases a slow intravenous drip of isoprenaline (Suscardia) or adrenaline may be necessary for a few hours to increase the strength of myocardial contraction and reduce peripheral vascular resistance.

When heart action is stable, the bypass cannulae are removed, the pericardium is partially closed, and the chest is closed with water-sealed drainage of the anterior mediastinum and the pericardial cavity.

Post-operative complications. The post-operative course after aortic valve surgery is usually smoother and convalescence is more rapid than after mitral valve replacement. This is because the lungs are less affected by aortic valve disease, and because the patients have usually not been in chronic cardiac failure for as long.

In the first few days post-operatively, ventricular extrasystoles are common. If these become more frequent than 10 per minute, treatment is required. The serum potassium level should be checked because hypokalaemia may cause this arrhythmia. The arterial P_{CO_2} should be measured because high P_{CO_2} levels can also provoke extrasystoles. If the serum potassium and the P_{CO_2} are normal, procaine amide should be administered intravenously at a rate of 100 mg./min. to a total dose of 1 g. A maintenance dose of 1 to 2 g. should be given in the intravenous drip over the subsequent 12 hours. Procaine amide lowers the blood pressure and this undesirable side effect must be watched while the drug is being given. Lignocaine has similar anti-arrhythmic properties and it is also used in the management of frequent extrasystoles and episodic tachyrhythmias (1 to 2 mg./kg. body weight given intravenously over several minutes, with a maintenance dose of 0·5 to 1·0 g. in 500 ml. over 8 hours).

Tricuspid Valve Disease

The tricuspid valve is never affected alone but approximately 10 per cent of patients with aortic and/or mitral valve disease have evidence of associated tricuspid valve lesions.

One-third of the patients with multi-valve disease have an incompetent tricuspid valve secondary to dilatation of the right ventricle. Correction of the mitral valve lesion results in a reduction in the size of the right ventricle and tricuspid valve function returns to normal. In the remainder, the tricuspid valve has been affected by rheumatic disease and valvuloplasty or replacement is required.

Haemodynamics

Stenosis of the tricuspid valve restricts the flow of venous blood from the right atrium to the right ventricle. Tricuspid incompetence allows a reflux of blood from the right ventricle into the right atrium during ventricular systole. Both lesions therefore cause enlargement of the right atrium and a hold up of the systemic venous return which produces engorgement of the systemic veins.

Symptoms and signs

The classical signs of tricuspid valve disease are due to overfilling of the systemic veins. Accentuated pressure waves may be visible in the jugular veins and enlargement of the liver occurs. The liver may even pulsate in cases of gross tricuspid incompetence. Tricuspid valve disease always occurs in association with mitral or aortic valve disease so that the patient also has symptoms and signs referable to malfunction of these valves.

Surgical treatment

Operation on the tricuspid valve requires heart-lung bypass and the mitral or aortic valve is repaired or replaced at the same time.

The valve is inspected through an incision in the right atrium. If the leaflets are normal and incompetence is due to stretching of the annulus secondary to right ventricular dilatation, plication alone may restore normality. In other cases, the valve leaflets show scarring and the valve requires replacement. A low-profile, disc type prosthetic valve is usually chosen for tricuspid replacement because the right ventricular cavity is usually not large enough to accommodate the caged ball type of valve. When suturing the valve in place, the surgeon must avoid inserting sutures in the region of the atrio-ventricular node and the bundle of His.

Multi-valve Disease

Approximately 25 per cent of patients with rheumatic valve disease require surgical replacement of more than one valve.

The operative procedure is technically more difficult and requires a longer period of heart-lung bypass than in single valve replacements but there are no additional specific problems in the post-operative management.

Because an adequate heart-rate is important to maintain cardiac output in the early post-operative period, pacemaker wires may be sutured to the right ventricle in theatre so that the heart can be paced at the optimum rate (90 to 100/min.) in the intensive therapy area.

CHAPTER 5

Congenital Heart Disease

Out of every thousand babies born, seven are liable to have a cardiac defect. Some defects are so severe that the baby dies shortly after birth, whereas others do not develop symptoms until childhood or adolescence. The nine commonest defects are listed in Table I.

TABLE I

Congenital Heart Disease

A classification of the nine congenital defects most commonly found in children who survive the first year of life

Defect	*Main effects*	*Percentage incidence*
Ventricular septal defect (VSD)	Left to right shunt	25
Patent ductus arteriosus (PDA)	Excessive pulmonary blood flow	12
Atrial septal defect (ASD)	Reduced systemic blood flow	12
Fallot's tetralogy	Right to left shunt	12
Transposition of great vessels	Usually reduced pulmonary blood flow	5
Tricuspid atresia	Cyanosis	2
Pulmonary stenosis	Obstructive lesions	9
Coarctation of aorta	Hypertrophy of left or	6
Aortic stenosis	right ventricle	5
Various uncommon defects	—	12

The causes of congenital heart disease are largely unknown. However, one important cause is widely recognised even among laymen: the heart develops during the first six weeks of intra-uterine life and maternal virus infections occurring at this stage of pregnancy are associated with a high incidence of congenital cardiac defects. The most harmful virus appears to be that of

German measles, but other viruses and certain drugs have also been implicated.

Defects which often cause death in the neonatal period or early infancy are transposition of the great vessels, large ventricular septal defects and severe pulmonary or aortic stenosis. Prompt diagnosis and emergency operation in these babies can be life-saving but full correction of the defect is not possible at the present time because heart-lung machines suitable for infants have not yet been properly developed. The surgeon does just enough to allow the baby to survive and grow, and a second definitive operation is performed later when the child is large enough to undergo open-heart surgery with heart-lung bypass.

Minor defects do not usually cause symptoms until late childhood or early adult life because they are compensated by ventricular hypertrophy and by adaptive changes in the pulmonary circulation.

The following are brief descriptions of the more common congenital heart defects.

Ventricular Septal defect (VSD)

This type of defect is usually about 1 cm. in diameter and it commonly lies at the top of the interventricular septum. It can be seen from the right ventricle under the 'septal' leaflet of the tricuspid valve (Fig. 19). From the left ventricle, the hole is seen just under the aortic valve. It causes a left to right shunt (arterial to venous) because the pressure in the left ventricle (120 mm. Hg) is greater than the pressure in the right ventricle (25 mm. Hg).

HAEMODYNAMICS

The natural history of VSD follows one of three patterns.

1. The largest group of patients have a moderate sized hole and develop symptoms in late childhood. These children are undersized and suffer from frequent chest colds (very like children with PDA). If left untreated, they may develop progressive obliterative pulmonary vascular changes leading to pulmonary hypertension.

2. A few patients (10 per cent) have a large defect more than 2 cm. in diameter and develop heart failure and pulmonary oedema in the first year of life. The powerful left ventricle ejects most of its blood through the defect and the blood passes into the lungs

together with the normal flow from the right ventricle. The lungs consequently become 'flooded'.

In these infants, the operation of 'banding the pulmonary artery' is done. In this operation a tape is tied around the pulmonary artery so as to narrow it and reduce the excessive blood flow into

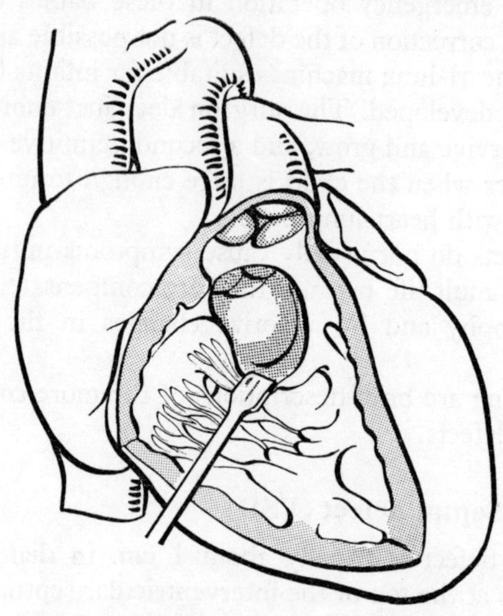

FIG. 19. Ventricular septal defect, viewed through the opened right ventricle. The chordae tendineae of the tricuspid valve are retracted aside. The cusps of the aortic valve can be seen through the defect.

the lungs. This is a 'temporising' operation and four or five years later, at a second operation, the band is released and the VSD is closed using heart-lung bypass.

3. About 20 per cent of patients have small VSD's which gradually close during the first 5 or 6 years of life and require no treatment.

SYMPTOMS AND SIGNS

Children with ventricular septal defects tend to be small for their age and subject to frequent respiratory infections. Those who develop pulmonary vascular changes show a gradual onset of exertional dyspnoea but, if the defect is small, symptoms may be slight. Large defects give rise to heart failure in infancy and temporising surgery may be required.

Diagnosis may be suspected if the child has a rough systolic murmur and thrill over the mid-precordium. X-ray screening shows excessive pulsation of the pulmonary arteries and engorgement of the pulmonary vasculature and both ventricles are usually slightly enlarged. Right heart catheterisation is usually required in order to confirm the diagnosis, and to measure the size of the left to right shunt.

SURGERY

Operation to close defects of moderate size is best undertaken between 5 and 10 years of age, using heart-lung bypass. The defect is exposed through the right atrium or ventricle and it is closed by suture if it is small or by a Dacron patch. The operative mortality is about 3 per cent.

The chief hazard of the operation is heart block, because the bundle of His runs along the lower edge of the hole, and it may be caught by the stitches. If there is any evidence of heart block on the ECG monitor in theatre, a wire, sewn to the apex of the right ventricle, is led to the surface of the chest so that artificial pacing can be commenced if heart block should occur. This wire is removed after 10 days if the patient's condition is satisfactory.

Patent ductus arteriosus (PDA)

The ductus arteriosus (Fig. 20) is a small channel, about 1 cm. in length, and just under 1 cm. in diameter (i.e. about the same diameter as the femoral artery) which runs from the main pulmonary artery to the underside of the arch of aorta. It functions in the foetus before birth when the lungs are collapsed and not in use. Blood pumped by the right ventricle into the pulmonary artery bypasses the lungs and goes through the ductus into the aorta to join the outflow from the left ventricle.

The ductus arteriosus has a sphincter-like muscle in its wall and normally closes within a few hours of birth. If it remains open, the baby has a 'persistent patent ductus arteriosus'.

In the foetus, blood flows from the pulmonary artery to the aorta but if the ductus remains patent after birth, the flow is reversed and blood passes from the aorta to the pulmonary artery. When the lungs expand after birth, the blood pressure in the

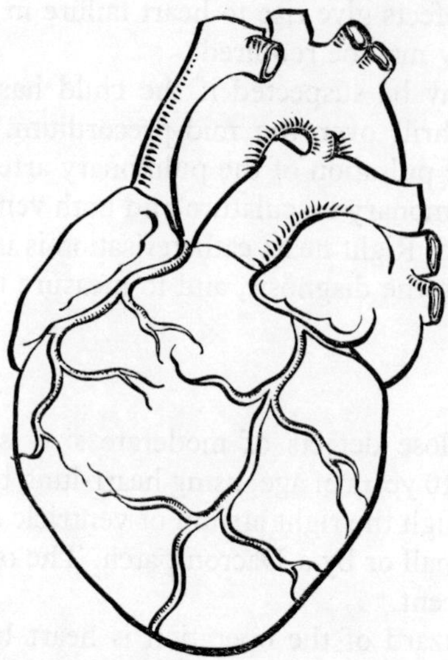

FIG. 20. Patent ductus arteriosus. This vessel runs from the underside of the aortic arch to the bifurcation of the pulmonary artery.

pulmonary artery falls to about 25/15 mm. Hg. Aortic pressure in the infant is 100/60, and blood therefore flows through the ductus from aorta to pulmonary artery as a left to right shunt. Like all left to right shunts, this has two main effects: (1) it reduces blood flow to the systemic circulation and (2) the pulmonary circulation is overfilled.

SYMPTOMS AND SIGNS

Children with a PDA are prone to repeated respiratory infections and tend to be undersized for their age. Most children are free from other symptoms until their late teens, but, if the ductus is a large one, heart failure may develop in infancy with severe congestion of the pulmonary circulation. Diagnosis is made by auscultation in the left infraclavicular region where the classical 'machinery' murmur can be heard.

X-ray screening usually shows engorgement of the pulmonary vasculature and excessive pulsation of the enlarged pulmonary arteries. Cardiac catheterisation will confirm the diagnosis if this is necessary, the principal finding on right heart catheterisation being an increase in the oxygen content of blood taken from the pulmonary artery.

SURGERY

Operation is usually performed at about 3 to 4 years of age, but may be undertaken earlier if severe pulmonary congestion or cardiac failure should appear. The operation is usually performed through a left thoracotomy and the ductus is ligated if it is less than 1 cm. in diameter. A wide ductus is divided between clamps with oversewing of the cut ends. The operative mortality risk is less than 1 per cent. There are no special post-operative problems but some mild elevation of blood pressure is common during the first few weeks. If the ductus is not closed surgically, these patients develop progressive obliterative changes in their pulmonary arteries which leads to pulmonary hypertension. Furthermore, as long as the ductus remains open there is a risk of sub-acute bacterial endocarditis (SBE).

Atrial septal defect (ASD)

There are several types of atrial septal defects, and the three commonest are illustrated in Figure 21. These defects are named according to the developmental abnormality which causes each. Whatever the cause, all atrial septal defects give similar signs and symptoms, and all require closure by open-heart surgery.

HAEMODYNAMICS

The principal effect of an ASD is an abnormal flow of blood from the left atrium into the right atrium, i.e., a 'left to right shunt'. This occurs because the pressure in the left atrium is normally 12 mm. Hg, whereas the normal right atrial pressure is only 5 mm. Hg. Blood flows into the right atrium through the defect to join the normal venous return from the superior and inferior venae cavae. The right ventricle has to cope with this extra blood and it hypertrophies. The pulmonary artery becomes dilated and the pulmonary circulation is overfilled with blood.

SYMPTOMS AND SIGNS

Children with defects in the atrial septum are usually free of symptoms until their late teens, but are more liable to develop chest colds than normal children. In their late teens they begin to ex-

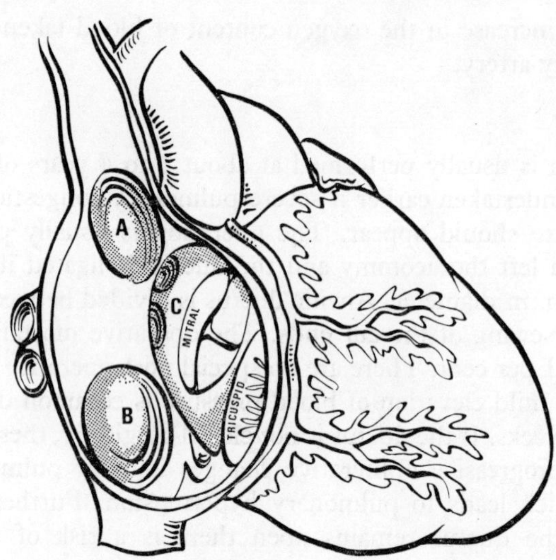

FIG. 21. Atrial septal defects. The three common types are shown through the opened right atrium: A a high secundum defect; B a foramen ovale defect; C an ostium primum defect which is often associated with a 'cleft' in the mitral valve.

perience exertional dyspnoea. If the defect is not closed obliterative changes develop in the pulmonary arteries because of the excessive flow and this leads in time (about 25 to 35 years) to pulmonary hypertension.

The diagnosis is suggested by a systolic murmur over the pulmonary artery, with a fixed delay in the closing sound of the pulmonary valve. The electrocardiograph usually shows the pattern of a right bundle branch block. X-ray screening shows an engorged pulmonary circulation, a dilated pulmonary artery with excessive pulsation and an enlarged right ventricle. The diagnosis is confirmed by right heart catheterisation which reveals that blood samples from the right atrium have an increased oxygen content.

SURGERY

Operative treatment involves closure of the hole using heart-lung bypass. A small defect less than 2 cm. in diameter can usually be closed with sutures; if the defect is larger, a patch of Dacron (Terylene) cloth is sewn over the hole. The operative mortality is about 3 per cent and the mortality rate rises with increasing age. Post-operative problems are similar to those occurring in any procedure involving bypass, together with cardiac arrhythmias such as atrial fibrillation or flutter. Arrhythmias may last for days or weeks but they usually respond to cardioversion or quinidine, and are not usually a cause for concern.

About 10 per cent of atrial septal defects have an associated defect called 'anomalous pulmonary venous drainage'. In this condition, some or all of the pulmonary veins join the right atrium instead of the left. This defect is remedied at operation by sewing the Dacron patch in such a way that the orifices of the abnormally placed pulmonary veins open into the left atrial side of the repaired septum.

In another 10 per cent of these cases there is an associated defect in the mitral valve. This takes the form of a slit or cleft in one leaflet which makes the valve incompetent and this slit must be repaired before the ASD is closed. Operation for this type of defect is associated with a higher operative mortality because stitches have to be placed close to the bundle of His and post-operative heart block is an occasional serious complication.

Fallot's tetralogy

This is the commonest cause of 'blue babies' who survive the first year of life. In the first year, transposition of the great vessels is commoner, but most babies with this defect die during the first few weeks or months after birth.

HAEMODYNAMICS

There are four cardiac defects which constitute the tetralogy (Fig. 22).

1. Pulmonary stenosis.
2. Ventricular septal defect (VSD).
3. Gross hypertrophy of the right ventricle.
4. The root of the aorta straddles the VSD.

The first two abnormalities are the important ones from a functional point of view. The pulmonary stenosis is usually valvular with, in addition, narrowing of the outflow tract of the right ventricle. Because of this stenosis, the right ventricle hypertrophies until it becomes more powerful than the left ventricle. Venous blood is pumped through the VSD into the left ventricle and thence up the aorta, i.e., it produces a right to left shunt. The patient therefore becomes 'blue' or cyanosed owing to the large amount of venous blood shunted into the systemic circulation.

SYMPTOMS AND SIGNS

Children with Fallot's tetralogy develop symptoms early in childhood and one-third of them die during the first year of life. The survivors suffer from 'cyanotic attacks' in which they become very blue and sometimes unconscious. These attacks are due to spasm of the abnormally thick muscle in the outflow tract of the right ventricle, i.e., the right ventricle strangles itself and blood flow to the lungs virtually ceases. All the venous blood from the venae cavae is pumped into the left ventricle and aorta and the child becomes darkly cyanosed. The immediate treatment of an attack is the administration of morphine and oxygen. Exertional dyspnoea and exertional intolerance are common symptoms.

Cerebral thrombosis is a common complication in children with

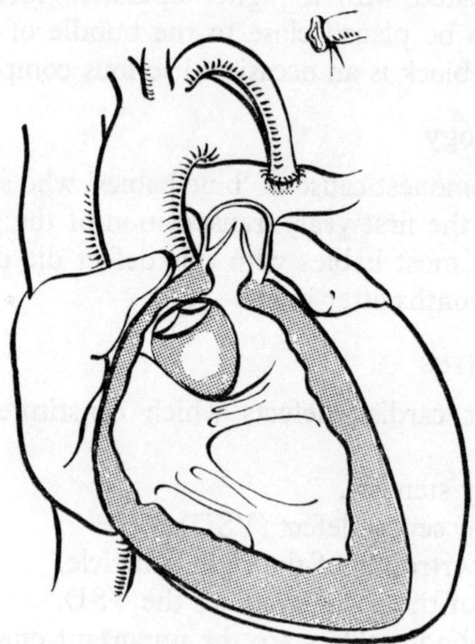

FIG. 22. Fallot's tetralogy: Blalock's operation. The diagram shows the defects of Fallot's tetralogy and also one of the palliative operations designed to lead more blood to the lungs.

Fallot's tetralogy. These children develop a polycythaemia (too many red blood cells) in an effort to compensate for the hypoxia which results from the right to left shunt, and their haemoglobin level is often 17 to 18 g./100 ml. (normal 13 to 15 g.). This makes the blood very viscous and liable to thrombose in the cerebral vessels.

Fallot's defects may be suspected in a cyanosed child whose ECG shows right ventricular hypertrophy. Right heart catheterisation and angiography are usually necessary to delineate the lesions.

SURGERY

Patients who have only a moderate degree of pulmonary stenosis and minimal cyanosis can wait until they are old enough and large enough to undergo complete correction of the defects. Operation is usually undertaken between 5 and 10 years of age on heart-lung bypass, a patch is inserted in the VSD and the pulmonary stenosis is cut and relieved.

Ill patients require a palliative operation to keep them alive and thriving and operation to correct the defects is postponed until they are older. The palliative operation is called Blalock's operation. It consists of making an anastomosis between the left subclavian artery and the left pulmonary artery (Fig. 22). The object of the operation is to circulate more blood through the pulmonary vessels in order to improve the degree of oxygenation. This operation does not require heart-lung bypass and is associated with relatively little risk although it is still a major procedure in very young cyanosed children. Post-operatively dehydration must be avoided because of the risk of cerebral thrombosis.

An alternative palliative operation consists of making a 'window' between the ascending aorta and the right pulmonary artery.

Transposition of the great vessels

Although this complex defect is one of the commonest found in new-born babies, it is usually incompatible with life and few children survive beyond the age of 1 year.

In this condition, the aorta arises from the right ventricle and the pulmonary artery from the left. The systemic and pulmonary circulations are therefore closed circuits unless there is a septal defect or patent ductus arteriosus through which mixing can occur.

SURGERY

Complete correction of the defect is not possible, but a near normal circulation can be achieved by a plastic procedure which alters the inter-atrial septum in such a way as to direct the venous blood from the right atrium to the left ventricle, and the oxygenated blood from the left atrium to the right ventricle. This complex operation requires heart-lung bypass and can only be done on children older than about 3 years.

In order that the child will survive until this operation can be carried out, a temporising operation is necessary. This consists of enlarging the foramen ovale to create a large atrial septal defect. This can be done in infants without opening the chest, as follows.

A cardiac catheter with an inflatable balloon at its tip (Rashkind) is passed from the saphenous vein up into the right atrium and through the foramen ovale into the left atrium. Under fluoroscopy, the balloon is inflated and pulled forcibly back into the right atrium. This tears the atrial septum and creates a defect.

Tricuspid atresia

In this rare condition the tricuspid valve has not formed, the right ventricle is vestigial, and the only exit for blood from the right atrium is through the foramen ovale into the left atrium. Children with this defect are darkly cyanosed and rarely survive the first few years of life.

SURGERY

Complete correction is not yet possible, but a significant degree of palliation can be achieved by Glenn's operation. In this procedure, the superior vena cava is anastomosed end-to-end to the right main pulmonary artery. This allows venous blood from the upper half of the body to reach the right lung where it is oxygenated, and the child becomes less cyanosed and able to lead a limited life.

Pulmonary stenosis (valvular)

In this condition the pulmonary valve is mal-developed and the cusps are stuck together leaving only a small orifice.

Pulmonary stenosis impedes the flow of blood out of the right ventricle, which hypertrophies in an effort to maintain a near-normal flow of blood to the lungs. The systolic pressure in the right ventricle consequently rises from a normal 20 mm. Hg to

80 or 100 mm. or even higher. If operation to relieve the stenosis is not undertaken, the right ventricle eventually fails and the patient dies.

SYMPTOMS AND SIGNS

A few cases of pulmonary stenosis are so severe as to cause right heart failure in infancy. In most patients, symptoms are few until late childhood or adolescence, when dyspnoea and occasionally angina of effort and syncopal attacks occur.

Diagnosis is suspected from the finding of a harsh systolic murmur over the pulmonary area and a palpably enlarged right ventricle. ECG confirms the right ventricular hypertrophy and X-ray screening shows an enlarged right ventricle, post-stenotic dilatation of the pulmonary artery, and translucent (avascular) lung fields. Right heart catheterisation reveals an elevation of pressure in the right ventricle with a gradient during systole across the pulmonary valve.

SURGERY

Operative treatment is performed on heart-lung bypass. The pulmonary artery is opened just above the valve and the valve is cut to give a normal opening. Operative mortality is about 1 per cent and there are no special post-operative problems.

Pulmonary stenosis (infundibular)

This condition is a narrowing of the outflow tract of the right ventricle and consists of a constriction at the 'neck' of the ventricle mainly as one of the principal defects of Fallot's tetralogy.

Coarctation of the aorta

This condition is dealt with on page 116.

Aortic stenosis

Congenital aortic stenosis used to be regarded as a relatively uncommon defect. However, it is now known that many cases of aortic stenosis diagnosed in adult life, which were formerly attributed to rheumatic fever, are in fact congenital in origin.

HAEMODYNAMICS

This is an insidious disease in which symptoms do not arise until secondary changes are very advanced. The left ventricle can maintain a near-normal flow through the narrowed valve for many years by immense hypertrophy. In doing so, however, the ventricular muscle may outstrip its coronary blood supply and sudden death from ventricular fibrillation is not uncommon in these cases.

SYMPTOMS AND SIGNS

The symptomatology of congenital aortic stenosis is similar to that of acquired rheumatic aortic stenosis (p. 39). Diagnosis depends on the demonstration of a systolic pressure gradient between the left ventricle and the aorta and angiography is necessary to distinguish whether the stenosis is valvular, sub-valvular or supra-valvular (see below).

SURGERY

Operation is performed with heart-lung bypass and the aorta is opened in order to inspect the valve. If rudimentary leaflets are present, incisions are made which will restore a normal opening without rendering the valve incompetent. In teenagers and adults the leaflets have usually become so deformed by the turbulent jet of blood coming through the narrow orifice, that replacement of the valve by a prosthesis or homograft is required. The mortality rate of operation for congenital aortic stenosis is closely related to the patient's age. It is less than 5 per cent in childhood, but rises to about 15 per cent if the condition is not discovered until middle age.

Of cases classified as congenital aortic stenosis, 15 per cent have the obstruction situated above or below the valve (supra-valvular and sub-valvular aortic stenosis).

Supra-valvular stenosis resembles a coarctation of the ascending aorta, the constriction being just above the aortic valve. This is relieved by inserting a patch to increase the diameter of the narrowed segment.

Sub-valvular aortic stenosis is usually due to a thick band of fibro-muscular tissue bulging into the outflow tract of the left ventricle just below the aortic valve. The obstruction can be relieved by cutting this band. A second type of sub-valvular aortic stenosis is unfortunately less amenable to existing surgical techniques. This type is called hypertrophic obstructive cardiomyopathy (HOCM) and the entire left ventricle is so abnormally muscular that it obstructs its own outflow during systole. There is no single band of muscle for the surgeon to cut, and an attempt is made to reduce the force of myocardial contraction by giving drugs such as propanolol (Inderal). Patients who do not respond to this treatment may be operated upon in the hope that division of some of the sub-valvular bands of muscle will relieve the obstruction, but the results of operation are usually disappointing.

CHAPTER 6
Heart Block

Heart block is a condition in which the atria and ventricles contract separately and at different rates owing to interference with the conducting system of the heart. Some knowledge of the anatomy and function of the conduction system is essential to an understanding of this condition (Fig. 23).

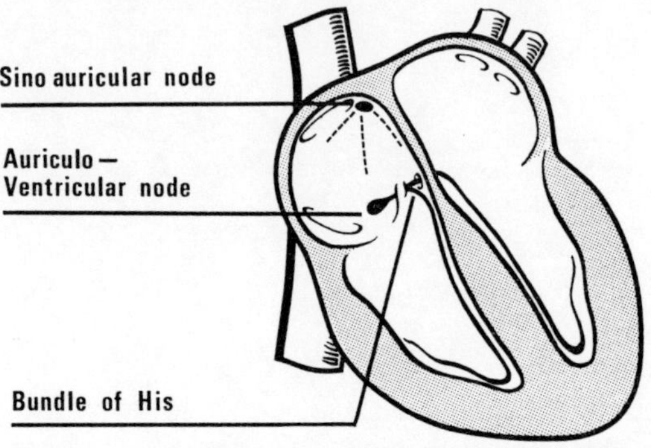

FIG. 23. The conduction system of the heart.

Each heart beat is initiated by the sino-atrial node (the 'pacemaker' of the heart) which generates an electrical impulse which spreads through the muscle of the atria and ventricles causing them to contract. The sino-atrial node is an area of the myocardium about 1 sq. cm. in size, which has the unique property of emitting regular electrical impulses. It lies in the angle between the superior vena cava and the right atrium.

As the signal passes through the atrial muscle it produces atrial contraction and the passage of this electric current appears as the P wave on an electrocardiogram tracing. This electrical impulse activates a second specialised portion of muscle situated at the bottom of the right atrium—the atrio-ventricular node. The signal is held up at this node momentarily, then it passes along the bundle of His to reach the ventricles. As the ventricles contract in response to the stimulus, the electrical changes are recorded as the QRS complex of the ECG.

If the bundle of His is damaged and not conducting, the signal from the sino-atrial node which reaches the A-V node cannot pass any further and the ventricles are cut off from the pacemaker, i.e., the patient has developed 'heart block'. The ventricles have their own inborn rhythmicity and continue to contract on their own but they do so at a very slow rate (about 30 to 40 beats per minute) and quite independently of the atria.

The diagnosis of heart block is made from the ECG (Fig. 24). This shows the atria beating normally (P waves), but infrequent ventricular beats (QRS waves) occur, quite unrelated to the P waves.

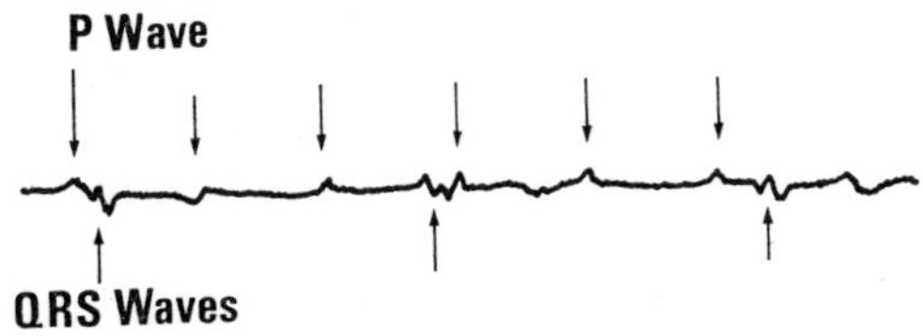

FIG. 24. Complete heart block.

Aetiology

The commonest cause of heart block is atherosclerotic occlusive disease of the coronary arteries. Many cases of heart block show occlusion of the coronary branches which nourish the bundle of His and the bundle has died and been replaced by a scar. A less common cause is myocarditis, either viral or diphtheritic. Approximately 10 per cent of cases are congenital in origin and a further small number result as a complication of cardiac surgery, where the bundle of His has been damaged by a stitch during the closure of a ventricular septal defect or in the course of aortic or tricuspid valve surgery.

Symptoms

The slow ventricular rate in heart block does not pump enough blood through the circulation to maintain normal bodily activity. Consequently, patients become chronically tired and listless and experience breathlessness after slight exertion. The classical symptom of heart block is the blackout or 'Stokes-Adams seizure'. During these attacks, the patient suddenly collapses, becomes unconscious and may have convulsions. The attack occurs because the ventricles do not contract for 5 to 20 seconds and the brain is the first organ to suffer—hence the blackout. Later in the disease, the heart muscle itself suffers because of the poor cardiac output, and heart failure follows, manifested as oedema, breathlessness, venous engorgement and enlargement of the liver.

Treatment

In 1954 an American surgeon, P. M. Zoll, suggested that a small electric current could be passed through wires attached to the ventricles so as to make them contract. This was the first conception of the artificial cardiac pacemaker. The modern unit comprises a set of long-life batteries powering an electronic device designed to send out small electrical impulses at a pre-set rate. The impulses are conducted to the ventricles by fine insulated wires, usually in the form of a cardiac catheter which ends in two platinum contacts (Fig. 25). The three pacemaker systems in common use are shown in Figure 26.

For temporary pacing, a pacemaker catheter is introduced into a vein at the elbow, then, under X-ray control, it is advanced until its tip reaches the apex of the right ventricle. The proximal end of the catheter has two terminals which are connected to the artificial pacemaker unit on the bedside locker. If the patient is ambulant, a miniature unit can be strapped to his wrist.

If the surgeon decides that the heart block is permanent and rrecoverable, the patient undergoes a small operation. A special pacemaker generator, encased in non-reactive material, is implanted under the skin in the axilla. Through a second incision in the neck, the pacemaker catheter is introduced into the external jugular vein and passed down to the heart under X-ray screening. The proximal end of the catheter is tunnelled down into the axilla to be connected to the generator unit.

When patients are to have an artificial pacemaker implanted, a temporary pacing catheter is first introduced via an arm vein under local anaesthesia. This is done as a precautionary measure in case the ventricles stop beating during anaesthesia for the implantation operation. The temporary catheter is left in place for a week after operation in case the jugular vein catheter of the implanted unit loses contact with the heart, i.e., the temporary catheter and bedside or 'wrist-watch' unit is retained as a stand-by for a week.

Two types of pacemaker are in common use, both as temporary units and as implantable units.

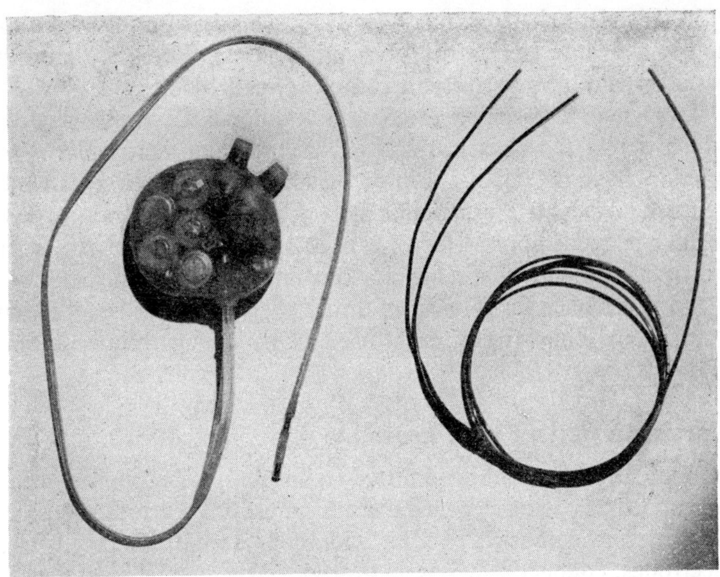

FIG. 25. Pacemakers. The photograph shows, on the left, an implantable endocardial pacemaker unit (Chardack-Medtronic), on the right an electrode catheter for temporary pacing.

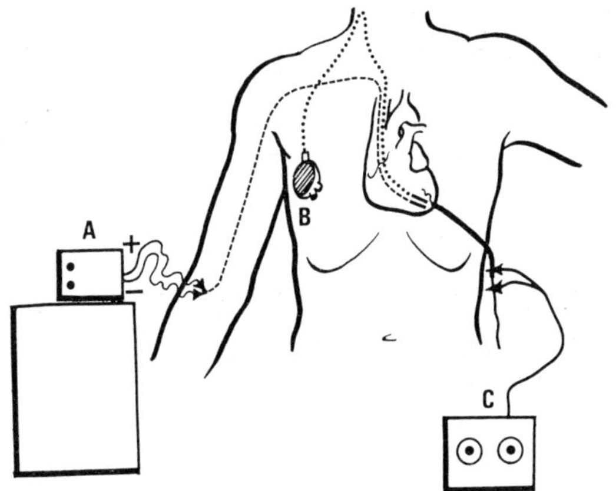

FIG. 26. Pacemakers. The systems commonly used for artificial cardiac pacing: A For temporary pacing, the pacemaker unit at the bedside is connected to a per-venous electrode catheter. B For permanent pacing the entire unit is implanted. C For emergency pacing, an external unit is connected to electrode wires which are introduced through a needle to the apex of the heart (Elecath).

1. 'Fixed-rate' pacemakers send out a pacing impulse continuously at whatever rate has been pre-selected. These are used in patients who have permanent complete heart block.

2. 'Demand' pacemakers contain additional electronic devices which detect the electrical activity arising from ventricular contraction (i.e., the QRS complex on an ECG). When a demand pacemaker detects a ventricular beat, it stops sending out its own regular pacing impulses for the space of one heart beat. In other words, if the patient's ventricles contract spontaneously, the demand pacemaker shuts itself off until the spontaneous heart action stops again. This type of unit is used for patients with intermittent or partial heart block.

Nursing a patient with heart block

As soon as the patient is admitted to hospital, a sterile emergency percutaneous pacing system ('Elecath') must be kept at the bedside. This system comprises a 5 in. wide-bore needle, insulated wire electrodes, connecting wires and a pacemaker unit. The patient is connected to an ECG monitor which will show the pattern illustrated in Figure 24. A temporary pacemaker should be introduced as soon as fluoroscopy can be arranged.

When the pacemaker is working properly, the ECG resembles the tracing shown in Figure 27. The important features of this

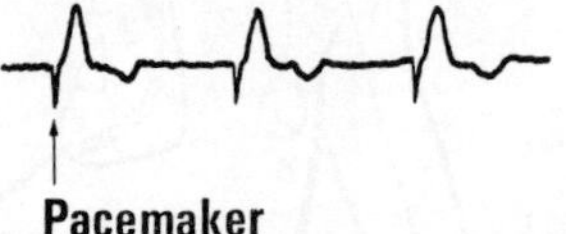

FIG. 27. The ECG in an artificially paced heart (see text).

tracing are the regularly occurring 'spikes' produced by the impulse generated by the pacemaker unit and the broadened QRS complexes due to the ventricular contraction which follows each pacemaker spike. If the pacemaker spike is not followed by QRS waves, the pacemaker is not working properly. The most likely cause is loss of contact between the electrode and the heart.

If this happens the nurse should confirm that pacing has stopped or has become intermittent by taking the patient's pulse. She should then switch on the temporary pacemaker and notify the doctor. Sometimes a change in the patient's position (e.g., turning him on to his right side) may let the heart move over enough to re-establish contact and normal pacing will be resumed. Usually, however, the patient must be returned to theatre and the electrode catheter repositioned. In the meantime, the temporary pacemaker system is used to maintain a safe heart rate.

If the heart fails to respond to a temporary pacing system, the electrical impulse may be too weak and the voltage should be increased by turning the control knob.

Fortunately, in the majority of cases, the ventricles resume beating at their own slow rate when pacing stops. The patient may suffer a blackout or a dizzy turn but he does not usually die. In the uncommon event of pacemaker failure in a patient who is not connected to a standby unit and in whom the ventricles do not resume beating spontaneously within one minute, the only course is to start external cardiac massage and ventilation of the lungs. This should be continued until a percutaneous emergency pacing system can be introduced by the doctor.

CHAPTER 7

Coronary Artery Disease

In common with other major arteries of the body, the coronary arteries may be affected by atherosclerosis. The right and left main arteries or their principal branches develop intimal thickening which leads to progressive narrowing and eventual thrombosis.

At the stage of stenosis, the blood flow (and hence the supply of oxygen) to the heart muscle is reduced. This may not cause symptoms for a long time but, as blood flow is progressively reduced, the patient is liable to experience exercise pain (cf. intermittent claudication) and finds that he develops chest pain after walking a certain distance or on climbing stairs—'angina of effort'. As the deficiency in circulation increases, he is liable to develop angina even at rest or when excited.

At any stage, either before the onset of symptoms or after the development of angina, coronary artery thrombosis may occur with a sudden and acute deficiency in blood supply to the heart muscle. This may have several results depending on the site and extent of the arterial block and on the efficiency of the collateral circulation which has developed during the stage of narrowing.

Sudden death may occur without warning due to the onset of ventricular fibrillation; blockage of a main artery may lead to death of the myocardium of most of one ventricle resulting in progressive heart failure or, if the patient survives, in cardiac aneurysm; interference with the blood supply of the conducting system of the heart may lead to heart block or other serious arrhythmias; a portion of heart muscle may become infarcted leading to replacement by fibrous tissue (myocardial infarct) and in favourable circumstances the patient will survive.

More than half of the patients who develop coronary thrombosis will survive provided that the early period of pain and shock is carefully managed and arrhythmias are prevented or treated promptly. In the event of cardiac arrest, full recovery is possible provided the patient is promptly treated.

Diagnosis

The diagnosis of coronary artery disease is made from clinical symptoms (e.g., angina) and is confirmed by the electrocardiogram. This shows a typical alteration in the ST segment in certain leads.

It is now possible to undertake coronary arteriography which will outline the diseased arteries and show the site and extent of the arterial changes (Fig. 28). It is usually reserved for patients in

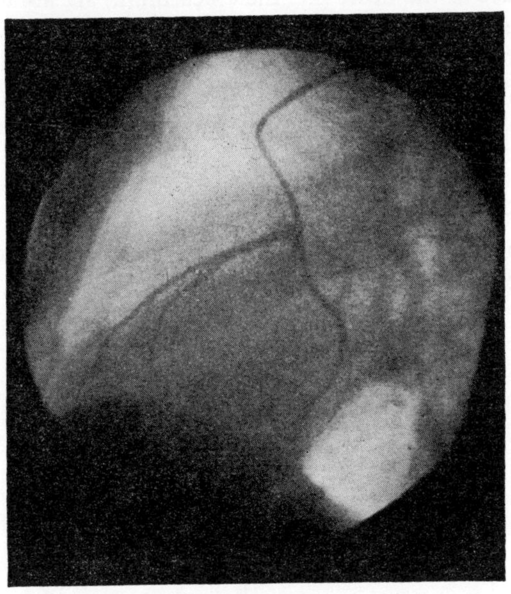

FIG. 28. A coronary arteriogram.

whom direct surgery of the coronary arteries (e.g., endarterectomy or bypass grafting) is under consideration.

Surgical treatment

At the present time, surgery for coronary artery disease is undertaken for the relief of severe angina or to improve blood supply to the myocardium when a future major occlusion seems probable. It has little to offer in the acute situation immediately after coronary thrombosis.

The immediate objective is to increase the blood supply to the myocardium. There are three ways of doing this: (1) the growth of small collateral vessels can be encouraged—Beck's operation, (2) extra blood can be brought in from outside the heart, e.g., Vineberg's operation, and (3) direct arterial surgery. The methods available for a direct surgical attack on the occluded segment are saphenous vein grafting or coronary endarterectomy.

BECK'S OPERATION

In this operation the inside surface of the pericardial sac and the outer surface of the heart (i.e. the epicardium) are abraded with a special instrument and sprinkled with asbestos powder. The object is to produce adhesions which will carry small collateral vessels and so improve the distribution of available coronary blood flow. This operation is now largely superseded by the more direct procedures outlined below.

VINEBERG'S OPERATION

In this operation (Fig. 29), the internal mammary artery is dissected free throughout most of its course as it runs down the inside

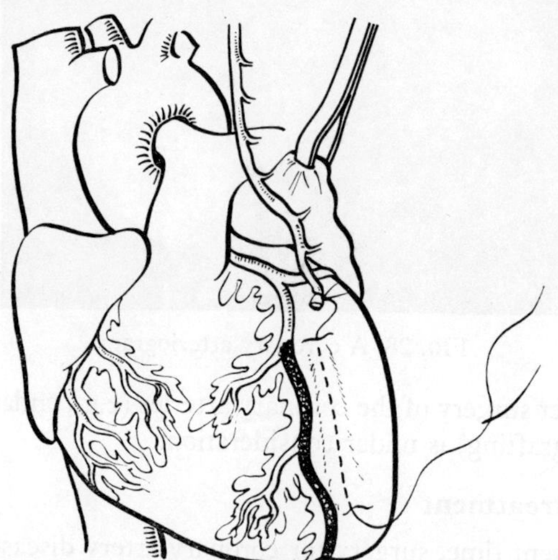

FIG. 29. Vineberg's operation: a tunnel has been made in the myocardium adjacent to a blocked coronary artery, and the internal mammary artery is drawn into it.

of the thoracic cavity close to the edge of the sternum. About 5 cm. of its distal end is implanted in a tunnel in the myocardium. It has been shown that numerous small vascular channels grow during the next six to nine months and connect the implanted artery to the coronary vascular bed.

DIRECT ARTERIAL SURGERY

Saphenous vein graft (Fig. 30). When a coronary angiogram shows that a main coronary artery is blocked in its first few centimetres but is patent beyond, it is possible to bypass the blocked segment with a vein graft. One end of the graft is anastomosed

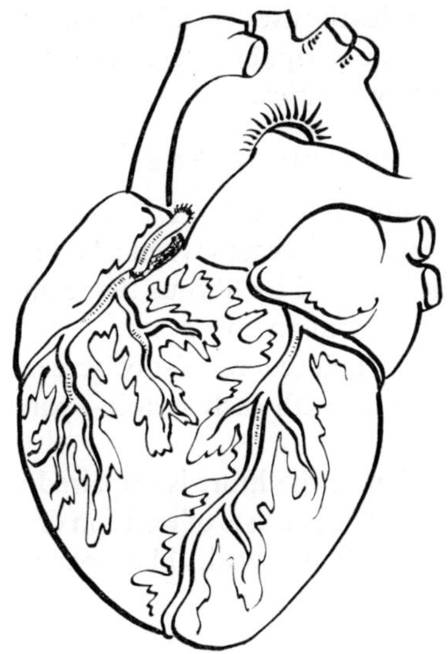

FIG. 30. A bypass graft: a short block in the right coronary artery has been bypassed by a a graft of saphenous vein.

to the ascending aorta the other to the side of the coronary artery beyond the block. Heart-lung bypass may be necessary during the fashioning of the anastomoses.

Coronary endarterectomy. Because of the relatively small size of the coronary arteries and the risk of re-thrombosis, endarterectomy is limited to the few patients who have a very short block in a main coronary artery which has a good calibre throughout the rest of its length. Heart-lung bypass is necessary for this form of coronary surgery.

Post-operative management

In addition to the usual complications which may follow thoracotomy, operations for coronary vascular disease are likely to be followed by dangerous arrhythmias and the patients usually have a low cardiac output for some days. The former calls for the use of anti-arrhythmic drugs such as procaine amide and lignocaine, and vigilant monitoring of the ECG. Facilities for D.C. defibrillation should be available by the bedside. A persistently low cardiac output due to myocardial failure carries a grave prognosis.

Management includes the use of mechanically assisted ventilation, drugs which reduce the peripheral vascular resistance and correction of acid-base abnormalities.

Myocardial Aneurysms

One of the less common sequels of coronary thrombosis is an aneurysm of the heart. This occurs when a large area of ventricular muscle has become replaced by fibrous tissue and the fibrous area gradually stretches to form an aneurysm.

The condition is diagnosed by X-ray screening which shows bulging of the aneurysm with each systole—paradoxical pulsation of the heart.

The pumping action of the heart is impaired and signs of heart failure appear. Treatment consists of excision of the weakened area and repair of the ventricular wall. The operation is done using heart-lung bypass.

CHAPTER 8

Post-operative Care

During the patient's illness, the heart and circulation have undergone adjustment to try and overcome the effects of the cardiac lesion. Operation terminates the need for these compensatory mechanisms and the heart and vascular system must readjust to the new haemodynamics. Post-operatively, the cardiovascular system may be unstable and care must be taken to anticipate or treat abnormalities which develop. Changes in heart action, peripheral circulation, acid-base balance (Appendix B) and fluid and electrolyte balance must be diagnosed and treated quickly.

All patients should be nursed in an intensive care area when they return from theatre. The length of stay depends on the type of operation performed and varies from 36 hours for an uncomplicated mitral valvotomy to a week or more for complex open heart operations.

The intensive care area is a place where a patient has the exclusive attention of a trained nurse aided by vital function monitors for 24 hours a day. These nurses should have special post-graduate training so that they can recognise complications as they arise.

Vital function monitors

These are the electronic machines which measure and display the various functions used to assess the patient's progress. The monitor usually consists of three parts: (1) the transducer which converts the physical function of temperature, blood pressure, heart rate, etc. into an electrical impulse; (2) the amplifier which magnifies this impulse and (3) the display which presents the measurement on a meter, a dial or an oscilloscope (Fig. 31).

The value of these monitors lies in their ability to make continuous measurements free from observer error without disturbing the patient. However, they must always be regarded as mere adjuncts to intelligent observation of the patient himself. The nurse must not become preoccupied with measurements to an extent which interferes with her equally important responsibilities of attending to the patient's mental and physical comfort. Recent psychological studies have shown that patients in intensive care

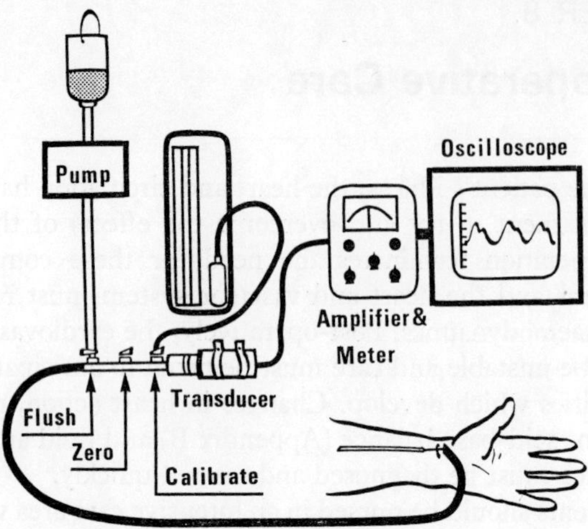

FIG. 31. A diagram of the equipment used to measure and display the arterial blood pressure from a fine cannula in the radial artery.

areas are prone to subtle psychological stresses and the harmful consequences of these stresses can be minimised or eliminated by a good nursing team.

Management of the patient in the intensive care area

Before an open-heart case returns from theatre, certain preparations should be made in the intensive care area:

1. The first 500 ml. of his i.v. fluid regime should be prepared: 5 per cent dextrose in water with the addition of 40 mEq. potassium chloride and antibiotics as ordered.
2. The vital function monitors should be switched on and calibrated ready to be connected to the patient.
3. The means of administering oxygen should be prepared and ready.
4. Drugs which are routinely necessary in the early post-operative period are drawn up in syringes and labelled, and drugs which may be required in emergency are assembled.
5. The D.C. defibrillator and resuscitation equipment is kept nearby.

The patient is particularly vulnerable in the period between leaving the operating theatre and being connected to the monitors in the intensive care area. The cardio-vascular system is particularly unstable at this time when the patient is awakening, perhaps re-establishing spontaneous breathing and beginning to move his limbs.

The transfer from theatre to the intensive care area should be supervised by the intensive care staff, and at least three trained nurses are required. They work as a team, each carrying out predetermined tasks, so that the patient arrives safely in the intensive care area, with his chest drainage re-established, his ECG displayed, and records of blood pressure, heart rate, etc. charted as quickly as possible.

The correct sequence of events when the patient arrives in the I.C.A. is as follows (Fig. 32).

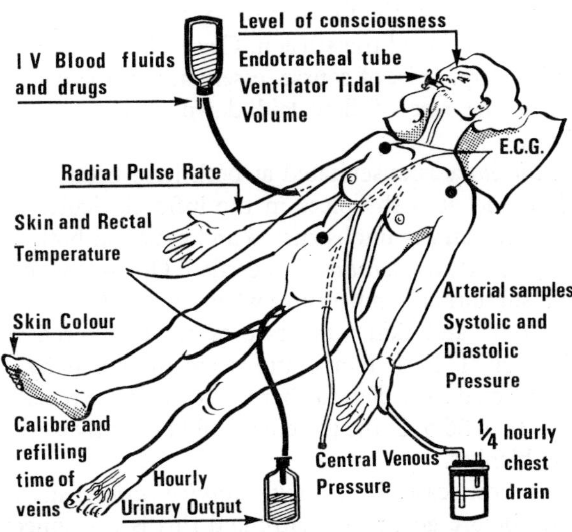

FIG. 32. A graphic representation of the vital functions which may be monitored after major cardiac surgery.

1. *Ensure a patent airway* with free movement of the chest on respiration. If mechanical ventilation is required, the anaesthetist connects the ventilator to the endotracheal tube. Alternatively, if the patient is breathing spontaneously, the anaesthetist puts on an *oxygen mask*.

2. Ensure that the *radial pulse* is readily palpable.

3. The *arterial cannula* is connected to the transducer and flushed, taking care to exclude air bubbles. A technician will then display the blood pressure on the monitor.

4. If there is no indwelling arterial cannula, the *blood pressure* is measured with a sphygmomanometer and charted.

5. *ECG electrodes* are applied and connected so that the technician can display the ECG and adjust the heart rate monitor.

6. *Chest drains* are connected to the water-sealed system, the tubing is 'milked' and the blood loss is charted.

7. The *intravenous drip* is re-established. Open-heart cases have a caval cannula introduced via the saphenous vein at the groin. The cannula is used to monitor the central venous pressure in theatre and in the intensive care area, and is also used as the route for fluid replacement. Open-heart cases have a second i.v. drip connected to a vein in the forearm or to the external jugular vein for the purpose of blood transfusion. Closed-heart cases have only the latter i.v. drip. It is, of course, essential that the correct fluids are given at the rate of flow laid down in the post-operative instructions.

8. The *air entry* is auscultated at both lung bases in the mid-axillary line and at both apices in the infra-clavicular region to ensure that air entry is unobstructed and equal on both sides.

9. The patient's *temperature* is recorded. Open-heart cases usually have a subnormal temperature when they return from theatre and both rectal and skin temperatures are monitored until the former is normal. Both temperatures are measured by thermocouples connected to an electro-thermometer. If the rectal temperature is less than 36·5°C, the patient should be gently warmed with an electric blanket.

10. Open-heart cases have a *self-retaining catheter* inserted into the bladder before going to theatre and this is re-connected to a closed, graduated reservoir on return to the intensive care area.

Common patterns in vital functions in the post-operative period

A change or trend in any of the vital functions in the early post-operative period may be the earliest indication of a potentially dangerous complication.

This section discusses the vital functions monitored in open-heart surgery with special reference to any changes which can occur and their significance.

BLOOD PRESSURE

This is the most important index of normal function of the cardiovascular system. A systolic blood pressure below 100 mm. Hg is a warning sign and, if the blood pressure falls below 80 mm. Hg for more than an hour, damage to the brain, kidneys, or heart conduction system is likely.

Hypotension. There are three basic causes of hypotension: (1) the heart is not pumping adequately, (2) there is insufficient blood in the circulation or (3) the peripheral blood vessels are abnormally dilated. In most cases, a combination of these factors is the cause of hypotension.

In the first 24 hours after cardiac surgery, the commonest cause of low blood pressure is an inadequate blood volume. Blood is transfused quickly, e.g. 200 ml. in 15 minutes, and if the blood pressure rises with this trial infusion, more blood is given slowly until the arterial pressure has returned to normal. If a rapid trial infusion does not produce a rise in blood pressure, the venous pressure must be checked.

If transfusion causes undue elevation of the venous pressure, the probable cause of hypotension is myocardial failure. This may be due to arrhythmia (too fast, too slow, or irregular beats) or to a primary weakness of the heart muscle. In either case, drugs are administered. Digoxin or propanolol are used to correct fast arrhythmias. A continuous drip of isoprenaline hydrochloride (Suscardia) may be given to increase the rate and force of myocardial contraction. A sinus bradycardia should be treated with atropine. Before these drugs are given, it is important to check that the acid-base balance and blood electrolytes are within normal limits, because acidosis or abnormal serum potassium levels are common causes of arrhythmia. Hypotension due to these causes can be corrected simply by giving sodium bicarbonate or potassium chloride.

One must remember that sedation can cause a fall in blood pressure which is not usually harmful. With pain and anxiety relieved, the patient stops producing large amounts of adrenalin and the subsequent vasodilatation allows the blood pressure to fall. The blood pressure also falls during sleep and this should be accepted as normal, provided that arousal of the patient (e.g., for physiotherapy) is associated with a rise in blood pressure.

If there is any doubt as to whether hypotension can be safely tolerated without intervention, the hourly urine output should be checked. If this is diminishing, action must be taken to raise the blood pressure without further delay.

Vasopressor drugs raise the blood pressure by causing vasoconstriction in some or all of the peripheral arterioles and venules. Some vasopressors also make the myocardium contract more strongly and increase the heart rate. The commonly used vasopressor drugs are metaraminol (Aramine), nor-adrenaline (Levophed), methylamphetamine (Methedrine), methoxamine (Vasoxine) and adrenaline. In cardiac patients, these drugs must not be used indiscriminately. They increase the work load of the heart because the rise in blood pressure is achieved by vasoconstriction and the peripheral resistance to blood flow is increased. Furthermore, the vasoconstriction may reduce the blood flow to the kidney and other organs and progressive kidney damage may occur despite a reassuringly normal blood pressure.

Hypertension. Abnormally high blood pressures are rarely seen after cardiac surgery, but they do occur in four well defined circumstances:

1. Essential hypertension. Patients with pre-operative essential hypertension have a raised blood pressure in the post-operative period. This high blood pressure is 'normal' for these patients and it rarely requires treatment.

2. Closure of a left to right shunt. When a patent ductus arteriosus, atrial septal defect or ventricular septal defect has been closed, the circulatory system adjusts rapidly to the new situation. The blood pressure is often higher than normal in the first week after operation but it falls to normal, without treatment, by the time the patient is able to go home.

3. Anxiety and pain. Many patients develop high blood pressure, tachycardia, and cold, pale hands and feet with empty superficial veins on their return to the I.C.A. This is due to vasoconstriction caused by excessive secretion of adrenaline and nor-adrenaline from the adrenal medulla. Reassurance and relief of pain by judicious sedation usually results in the blood pressure returning to normal and the hands and feet warm up as the circulation improves.

It is important to be able to distinguish the peripheral vasoconstriction caused by hypovolaemia—low blood volume. If analgesics and sedatives are given to a patient with hypovolaemia in a dosage high enough to cause vasodilatation, a dangerous fall in blood pressure will result.

4. Hypoxia. A sudden rise in blood pressure post-operatively is often due to hypoxia. The probable causes are upper airway obstruction (e.g., crusting of an endotracheal or tracheostomy tube) or atelectasis. These complications should be looked for and the arterial oxygen measured. Treatment lies in correction of the cause.

Patients attached to a mechanical ventilator may show a sudden rise in blood pressure for similar reasons. Hypertension in these patients suggests that the ventilator settings are wrong, or that the patient requires further sedation so that he will accept the mechanically controlled breathing.

Central venous pressure (normally 5-10 cm. water above mid-thorax). This is measured through a cannula introduced into the inferior vena cava via the saphenous vein or in the superior vena cava via the external jugular vein. Venous pressure is measured on a column of dextrose-water or saline and the centimetre scale is adjusted so that zero on the scale is at the same horizontal level as the patient's heart. When the venous cannula is connected to the saline column, the level of saline represents the central venous pressure (in centimetres of water). Patency of the cannula can be checked by asking the patient to cough or by pressing on his abdomen, because each produces a brief rise in central venous pressure. The cannula is also used for the intravenous drip and it therefore does not clot between readings of the venous pressure. High concentrations of powerful drugs should not be given in this drip, because an excessive dose could be given inadvertently when the venous pressure was measured.

A low central venous pressure usually indicates that the patient has a low blood volume. It suggests that blood replacement has been inadequate, and more blood should be given until the venous pressure is normal. In babies and young children, a low central venous pressure can also be due to dehydration and the venous pressure is a useful guide to fluid intake in the post-operative period.

A high central venous pressure may be a sign of over-transfusion, but there are many other factors which can raise the venous pressure and a high central venous pressure is not a bar to further transfusion. During the first 12 hours after operation, a central venous pressure of between 10 and 20 cm. of water is quite common. This may be due to peripheral vasoconstriction which shifts blood into the central venous pools, to a non-compliant muscular right ventricle in cases of ASD and pulmonary stenosis, or to a degree of right heart failure in cases with pulmonary hypertension or long standing valvular disease. Intermittent positive pressure ventilation also raises the central venous pressure by 2 or 3 cm. because the normally negative pressure within the chest is converted to a positive pressure during mechanical inflation of the lungs. A high central venous pressure is one of the signs of cardiac tamponade (p. 85).

TEMPERATURE

When the patient returns from theatre, his temperature is often subnormal and an electric blanket should be switched on until his rectal temperature is 37°C. Thereafter, only the lightest of bed covers are required, provided the room temperature is not lower than 19°C. On the first and second post-operative days, the patient's skin temperature often rises to 38°C or even 39°C.

This pyrexia is not necessarily due to infection. It is more usually caused by the transfusion of large amounts of homologous blood, by pyrogens derived from the extra-corporeal circuit, or by a mediastinal haematoma. If the temperature is still elevated on the third or fourth day, infection is the probable cause.

A high temperature does not benefit the patient and, indeed, it is harmful because it increases oxygen consumption and the work load of the heart. If the skin temperature rises above 38°C during the first 36 hours after operation, blankets should be removed and, if it rises above 39°C, the patient should be tepid sponged.

HEART RATE

Tachycardia is normal after cardiac surgery and a heart rate of 110 per minute is acceptable. Faster rates may accompany a rise of temperature or be due to auricular fibrillation. A steadily rising heart rate, with a steady temperature and respiratory rate is suggestive of hypovolaemia, and the rate of blood loss from the chest drains should be checked.

A sudden change in heart rate usually signals the onset of an arrhythmia.

In the I.C.A. the nurse should count the heart rate at the apex and the radial pulse. Where these differ (e.g. in auricular fibrillation) both rates should be charted.

RESPIRATORY RATE

The normal adult respiratory rate is 16 to 18 per minute. After thoracotomy the rate increases because the patient takes smaller breaths to avoid pain in his wound.

A *rising* respiratory rate is usually due to hypoxia caused by poor aeration of the lungs consequent upon blockage of a bronchus by mucus, or compression of the lung by a haemothorax. When the patient has a tracheostomy, tachypnoea may be due to obstruction of the tracheostomy tube.

An abnormally *slow* respiratory rate (less than 15 per minute) is uncommon in the post-operative period. The probable cause is excessive sedation and a slow respiratory rate may lead to a dangerous degree of carbon dioxide retention (Appendix B).

URINE OUTPUT

The best guide to renal function in the post-operative patient is the volume of urine secreted. Renal dysfunction is not uncommon in patients with severe heart disease and a careful check on the urinary output is an important part of post-operative management.

Urine is drained by the catheter to a closed measuring cylinder and the volume secreted is charted every hour. When renal function is normal, the hourly output depends on the patient's fluid intake and a normal daily intake of 2·5 litres should produce an output of at least 50 ml. per hour. An output of less than 30 ml. per hour calls for vigilance, and an output of less than 20 ml. per hour requires active and prompt treatment.

Oliguria may be due to inadequate fluid intake and, in these circumstances, the concentration of urea in the urine is normal or raised. In most patients, however, oliguria has an ominous significance and indicates incipient renal failure. This could be due to hypotension, hypovolaemia, incompatible blood transfusion or an adverse reaction to a drug. A much rarer cause is blockage of a renal artery by embolus.

When signs of renal dysfunction are recognised early, further damage can usually be averted by inducing a brisk diuresis with 80 to 200 mg. of frusemide (Lasix) given intravenously.

After heart-lung bypass, the urine output is usually copious for 6 to 12 hours and it is not uncommon for 500 ml. per hour to be voided during this time. This represents the excretion of the large volume of fluid used for priming the heart-lung machine. Following this early high output, hourly urine volume falls to 30 to 50 ml. during the subsequent 12 hours. Thereafter, the output should increase again provided the patient's fluid intake has been adequate.

CHEST DRAINS

The thoracic cavity is almost invariably drained after thoracotomy because bleeding would otherwise produce a haemothorax which would compress the heart and lungs.

All chest drains are connected to a reservoir by airtight tubing in such a way that fluid can get out of the thoracic cavity but air cannot be sucked in. The simplest chest drainage system (Fig. 33)

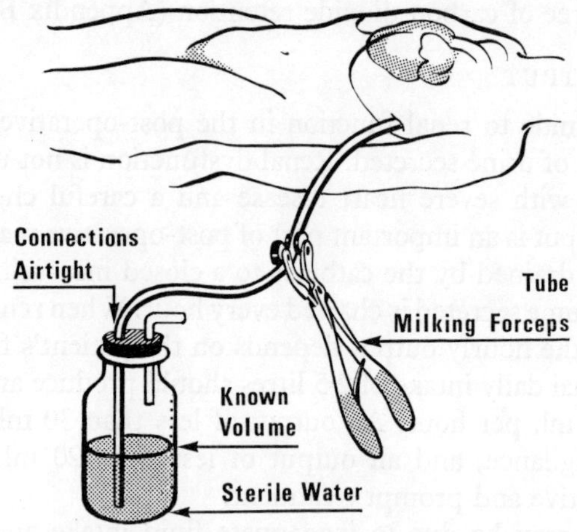

FIG. 33. A simple form of water-sealed chest drain.

leads the tube under water in the collecting bottle—a water-seal drain. This prevents the entry of air into the tube and hence into the chest but it is essential to keep the drainage bottle more than 18 in. lower than the patient, otherwise water could run into the thoracic cavity.

Most chest drainage systems have a water seal, a graduated reservoir to measure the amount of blood loss, and suction to help evacuation of blood from the chest. Disposable units are now used in most centres.

The three cavities in the chest which require to be drained are the pleural cavity, the mediastinum and the pericardium. In mitral valvotomy, a left thoracotomy is used and only the left pleural space is drained. In most open-heart operations, the approach to the heart is through a median sternotomy and it is usual to drain the anterior mediastinum and the pericardial cavity with separate tubes.

The nurse's responsibilities for chest drains are three-fold:

1. She must ensure that all connections in the system are airtight.

2. She must 'milk' the tube as it emerges from the chest to prevent clotting of blood in it. The tubing should be milked vigorously at least once every 10 minutes for the first 12 hours—less frequently thereafter. This is best done with the instrument shown in Figure 33.

3. She should chart the volume of blood lost through the drains every 15 minutes.

If there is any suspicion of a leak in the chest drainage system, the tubing is clamped immediately close to the chest wall and a doctor is notified. Suitable forceps should be kept beside the drainage system.

BLOOD LOSS AND REPLACEMENT

It is essential to maintain the patient's blood volume as near normal as possible after operation. A 'blood balance' chart is kept, and the volume of blood lost through the drains and the volume transfused are noted every 15 minutes for the first 12 hours.

The rate at which blood should be given depends on a number of factors which must be assessed together. As a general rule the amount of blood given should exceed that lost through the chest drains by about 20 per cent. When blood is being transfused rapidly, the venous pressure must be closely watched because a sustained rise in response to transfusion suggests either that too much blood has been given, or that the heart is failing. Before each new bottle of blood is connected to the i.v. line, the nurse should check carefully that its label bears the patient's name, and address, hospital number and blood group.

FLUID AND ELECTROLYTE BALANCE

For 12 to 24 hours after open-heart surgery with bypass, paralytic ileus is present and attempts at oral feeding result in abdominal distension and vomiting. The patient's fluid requirements must be given by the intravenous route. The amount of fluid administered can be critical because too much could cause pulmonary oedema and too little could lead to renal dysfunction.

An intake-output chart is charted hourly. The volume and composition of the intravenous fluids will be prescribed and the nurse must ensure that the intravenous drip rate is adjusted so that the correct volume is given in the correct period of time. If the intake falls behind, it is dangerous to try and remedy this by abruptly increasing the drip rate because this could precipitate pulmonary oedema. The correct procedure is to make up the deficit slowly during the next few hours.

The only serum electrolyte level which is significantly changed by major cardiac surgery is that of potassium and it is usually necessary to add potassium chloride (1 g. = 13 mEq.) to the intravenous fluids in order to maintain normal potassium levels.

In most patients, oral fluids and feeding can be commenced 24 hours after surgery. Patients who still require mechanical ventilation must be given fluid, electrolytes and calories by intra-gastric drip. Patients with persistent paralytic ileus must continue to receive fluids etc. by the intravenous route, and, after the first 24 hours, the patient's intake should include electrolytes, calories and vitamins.

OXYGEN THERAPY

Impaired pulmonary function occurs in many types of heart disease and thoracotomy and heart-lung bypass produce further impairment of ventilation. The concentration of oxygen breathed by the patient must be increased post-operatively in order to avoid hypoxia. After closed mitral valvotomy and after open-heart surgery in children and young adults, oxygen therapy is required for only 4 to 12 hours. In cases of valve replacement and in older patients, oxygen therapy is often necessary for several days.

The best method of giving oxygen is by using a disposable plastic mask and two types are shown in Figure 34. Oxygen tents are now rarely used except in paediatric and neonatal units, because they are inefficient for adult patients and interfere with the nursing of the patient. They also constitute a major fire hazard.

The Pneumask, with an oxygen flow of 6 to 10 litres per minute, gives the patient an oxygen concentration of 60 to 80 per cent and it should not be used with oxygen flow rates of less than 5 litres per minute. If low flow rates are used, the space between the mask and face is not flushed with oxygen between breaths, and the patient inhales some of the carbon dioxide which he has just breathed out.

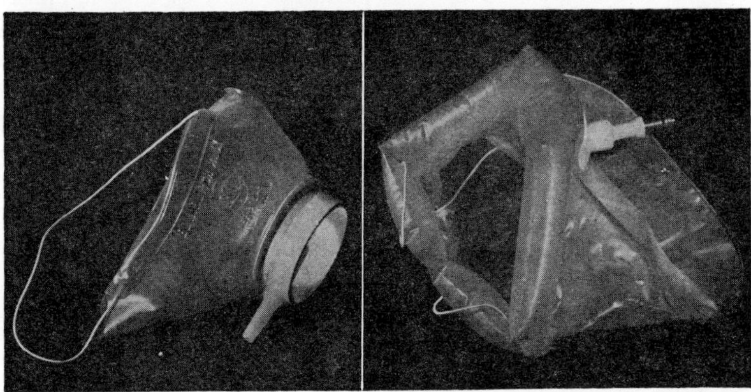

FIG. 34. Oxygen masks: the 'Edinburgh' mask on the left and the 'Pneumask' on the right.

This could quickly lead to a build-up of carbon dioxide causing drowsiness, coma and even death.

The 'Edinburgh' venturi mask, with an oxygen flow of 2 to 6 litres per minute, gives inhaled oxygen concentrations of 25 to 40 per cent. Light tubular extensions can be added to this mask to increase the oxygen concentration to 60 per cent.

Patients suffering from chronic bronchitis should not be given high concentrations of oxygen because the respiratory centre of these patients has become accustomed to work under hypoxic conditions and raised carbon dioxide levels. The administration of high concentrations of oxygen removes the hypoxic stimulus and may cause apnoea.

The amount of oxygen necessary can be checked by measurement of the oxygen content of arterial blood samples. These are usually withdrawn from an indwelling arterial cannula so as to avoid repeated arterial puncture. (See Appendix B.)

ARTIFICIAL VENTILATION

Some patients are too ill or too weak to breathe adequately after operation and they require mechanically assisted ventilation. All the ventilators in common use have the same basic function. They blow oxygen or air into the patient's lungs with little or no effort required from the patient. They are used with an endotracheal or tracheostomy tube or, rarely, with a tightly fitting face mask. Their controls regulate the concentration of oxygen as well as the volume, pressure and frequency of each respiration. Some machines are 'patient triggered', i.e., they only inflate the lungs in response to an inspiratory effort from the patient. Others are 'automatic' and deliver gases according to their setting, irrespective of the patient's own efforts. With the latter type, the patient can be heavily sedated, in the knowledge that his ventilation is being regulated by the machine.

It is important not to allow a patient to breathe 'in competition' with a mechanical ventilator. This can occur when the patient is anxious and undersedated, when the ventilator is not delivering the amount of oxygen he requires, or when it is not washing out sufficient carbon dioxide.

If a patient connected to a mechanical ventilator makes respiratory efforts asynchronously with the machine, the doctor should be notified immediately.

TRACHEOSTOMY

Tracheostomy is an operation whereby an opening is made into the trachea at the base of the neck to facilitate breathing and the airway is kept patent by a tube inserted directly into the trachea.

After cardiac surgery, there are three groups of patients who may require tracheostomy. (1) Patients who require mechanical ventilation for several days because of impaired lung function or because of the severity of their illness. (2) Patients who cannot cough effectively and so retain bronchial secretions which are liable to plug the bronchi or become infected. A tracheostomy allows periodic bronchial suction to be performed. (3) Patients who have developed respiratory obstruction due to oedema or inflammation of the upper respiratory passages and vocal chords.

Two types of tube commonly used in tracheostomies are shown in Figure 35. Inflatable cuffs serve two purposes: they make the airtight fit necessary for mechanical ventilation and they prevent

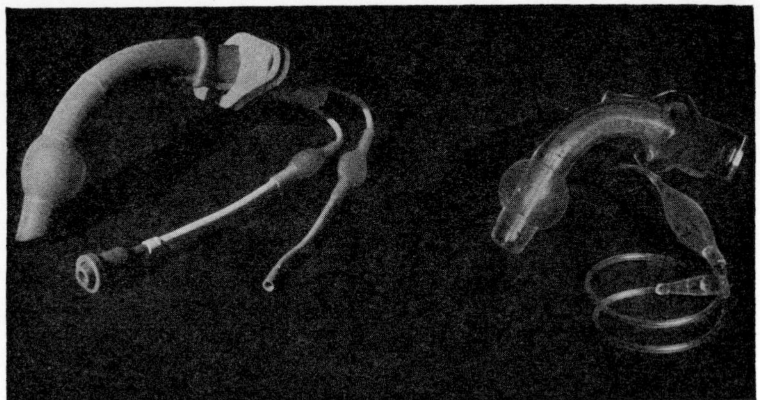

FIG. 35. Tracheostomy tubes: the tube on the left has two cuffs which are inflated alternately to alter the site of pressure on the tracheal lining.

secretions from the oro- and naso-pharynx from trickling down into the trachea and bronchi.

Management. Nursing a patient with a tracheostomy calls for extra watchfulness, scrupulous asepsis, and gentleness in handling the tube. The tube should be changed every 24 hours and the inflatable cuff should be released for 5 minutes every 2 hours in order to prevent compression necrosis of the tracheal lining. Aspiration should be performed with a soft whistle-tipped catheter connected to a source of high flow–low pressure suction (100 mm. of Hg negative pressure). The base of the catheter should be kinked to cut off the suction while it is being passed down the trachea as far as it will go and suction is maintained as the catheter is slowly withdrawn. The catheter should not be pushed and pulled up and down the trachea because this has a very delicate epithelial lining which is easily damaged and bleeds readily.

It is not possible to make rules about the frequency of aspiration. This depends on the amount of secretion present which varies from patient to patient and from day to day in the same patient. Aspiration every two hours is usually sufficient but it should also be performed every time the cuff is deflated or when secretions can be heard to bubble in the trachea or tracheostomy tube.

Air entering the air passages is normally warmed and humified as it passes through the nose and pharynx, but this mechanism is lost during tracheostomy. Provision must be made to humidify the air or oxygen breathed.

The nurse should know how to detect partial blockage of a tracheostomy tube. This is usually obvious when secretions are copious because they dry and encrust the tip of the tube. Partial blockage is not so easily recognised. When a patient is breathing spontaneously, the signs of partial blockage are restlessness, over-action of the respiratory muscles, a rise in pulse rate and temperature, and usually a rise in blood pressure. If the patient is connected to a mechanical ventilator, an increase in inflation pressure may be the first sign of partial blockage. Patency of the tube can easily be tested by passing a suction catheter and, if there is any difficulty passing it beyond the tip of the tracheostomy tube, partial blockage should be suspected and the tube should be changed.

CHAPTER 9

Post-operative Complications

Every organ in the body depends on the integrity of the circulation for its supply of oxygen and for the removal of metabolic products, and any malfunction of the cardio-vascular system is liable to be followed by progressive damage in other organs. This damage may itself affect heart action and a vicious circle is produced. For this reason, it is important to detect and treat complications after cardiac surgery without delay. Since the nurse spends most time with the patient in the post-operative period, she can detect the earliest signs of a serious or life-threatening complication, provided she has been trained to recognise and interpret the signs correctly. In this chapter, the common complications which can occur in the post-operative cardiac patient are described in detail.

Haemorrhage

Haemorrhage is more common after cardiac surgery than after major surgery elsewhere in the body for two reasons: (1) the normally negative pressure within the thoracic cavity encourages the continuance of venous oozing; (2) the use of heart-lung bypass depletes the blood of certain clotting factors and so interferes with the normal haemostatic process.

However, both the pericardial and pleural cavities can be drained to water-sealed collection systems, and the rate and total blood loss can be measured and replaced. Provided that all the blood is evacuated from the chest, and the volume lost is replaced, the patient's condition will not deteriorate. Difficulties occur only when the drains are inefficient or when blood is allowed to clot in the drain or in the mediastinum, pericardium or pleural spaces. In these closed areas a few hundred millilitres of blood can press on the heart or lungs and lead to rapid deterioration of the patient's condition.

Cardiac tamponade

This is a condition in which blood or clot in the pericardial sac progressively compresses the relatively soft atria and great veins.

It results in a progressive fall in blood pressure with a reduction in pulse pressure, a rise in heart rate and in central venous pressure. The patient becomes anxious and restless and the respiratory rate rises. Cardiac tamponade is a dangerous complication and the patient must go back to theatre, so that blood and clot can be evacuated from the pericardium and the source of bleeding stopped.

Haemothorax

Haemothorax is a condition in which blood or clot collects in the pleural cavity. It is commonest in those who have had a second thoracotomy. In these patients, adhesions which formed between the lung and chest wall after the first operation are divided to gain access to the heart, and blood tends to clot on the resulting raw areas before it can reach the chest drain. This collection of blood in the pleural cavity causes compression and collapse of the underlying lung, which becomes airless. The loss of functioning lung tissue causes the respiratory rate to rise and the patient may become cyanosed or require oxygen to keep his arterial P_{O_2} at a safe level.

The presence of a haemothorax can be confirmed by X-ray (Fig. 36). If the blood is still fluid, it can be aspirated through a wide-bore needle but, if clotting has occurred, the patient must return to theatre for evacuation of the clot.

Atelectasis

Atelectasis is collapse of part or the whole of a lung. It may be due to compression by a haemothorax but absorption collapse due to blockage of a bronchus by secretion is commoner.

Patients after thoracotomy do not breathe as deeply as normally nor do they cough effectively because of pain, oversedation or the presence of an endotracheal tube. Consequently the normal bronchial secretions are retained and may block a small or large bronchus. The affected area of lung is no longer ventilated, the air in it is absorbed into the pulmonary capillaries and the alveoli collapse. Blood still flows through the pulmonary capillaries of the collapsed segment of lung, but it can no longer take up oxygen and so leaves the lung as unoxygenated 'venous' blood.

Atelectasis lowers the oxygen content of the blood in the systemic arteries, and, if the area of collapse is large enough, cyanosis will result. The occurrence of atelectasis is diagnosed by auscultation and confirmed by X-ray (Fig. 37).

It is treated in the first instance by encouraging deep breathing and coughing, or if the patient's trachea has been intubated, by bronchial suction. If this fails to dislodge the causal plug of mucus, bronchoscopy and direct vision bronchial toilet is necessary.

Cerebral complications

Although cerebral complications are uncommon after cardiac surgery, air embolism of the cerebral arteries can occur after open-heart operations, and thrombus embolism of the cerebral arteries may occur in those who have thrombus in the left atrium, e.g., during mitral valvotomy.

Air embolism is one of the most dreaded complications associated with open-heart surgery. During operations with heart-lung bypass, some chambers of the heart are inevitably filled with air during the intracardiac part of the operation. When the incision in the heart has been closed, great care must be taken to vent it of air before the heart takes over the circulation again. Any air which is left in the left side of the heart will be swept out into the aorta when ventricular action resumes, and may pass up the carotid or vertebral arteries to block some of the smaller cerebral arteries. When this happens, the patient will be slow to regain consciousness when he returns to the intensive care area and signs of paralysis will become evident during the next few hours.

Less commonly, the air bubble remains trapped in the heart (sometimes in the left atrial appendage) and it is released into the systemic circulation an hour or so later when the patient is moved or propped up.

Thrombus embolism occurs as a complication of closed mitral valvotomy. About 12 per cent of patients who undergo operation have thrombus in the left atrium, and this may be dislodged by the surgeon's finger as it enters the heart, thus forming a systemic embolus. The commonest site of impaction of an embolus from the heart is in the cerebral circulation, because the innominate and carotid arteries are the first large branches of the aorta. The signs of cerebral thrombus embolism are similar to those seen after air embolism, i.e., the patient remains unconscious or drowsy and paralysis develops.

The management of cerebral embolism due to either air or clot consists of measures to reduce the cerebral oedema which develops during the 12 to 24 hours after blockage of a cerebral artery. Mannitol (20 g. in 100 ml.) is given through a caval drip and the dose is repeated two hours later. If the patient is unconscious or if the cough reflex is affected, tracheostomy should be performed. If the patient is deeply unconscious, mechanical ventilation may be necessary. Mannitol induces a profuse diuresis and the bladder should always be catheterised and continuous drainage established. In addition, the nursing procedures which are required for unconscious patients should be implemented, i.e., regular turning, physiotherapy and intra-gastric drip feeding.

In most cases the prognosis is good and signs of recovering function can be expected after 36 to 48 hours. Many patients regain almost normal function.

Post-operative psychosis

Many patients who undergo major cardiac surgery exhibit signs such as mild hallucinations, disorientation or paranoia in the early post-operative period. The patient may become obstreperous and difficult to control and he may detach his monitoring leads and i.v. drips. Several factors probably interact to produce this syndrome, but the principal cause seems to be the physical and mental stresses affecting an ill patient in an intensive care area. Treatment is symptomatic and consists in careful sedation and reassurance, bearing in mind that any degree of hypoxia will worsen symptoms of cerebral dysfunction. The incidence of post-operative psychosis can be reduced by modifications in the management of intensive care areas designed to keep the patient in touch with the outside world.

Systemic embolism

In some cases of closed mitral valvotomy, thrombus may be dislodged from the left atrium and block one of the systemic arteries. The commonest site of impaction is the brain and the next most common is in the arteries to the lower limb. If embolism has occurred in theatre, one leg will be pale, cold, and pulseless at the end of operation, and immediate embolectomy should be undertaken.

Less commonly, thrombus breaks off from the left atrium during the early post-operative period. Impaction of this embolus in the iliac or femoral arteries causes pain in the leg. The distal pulses

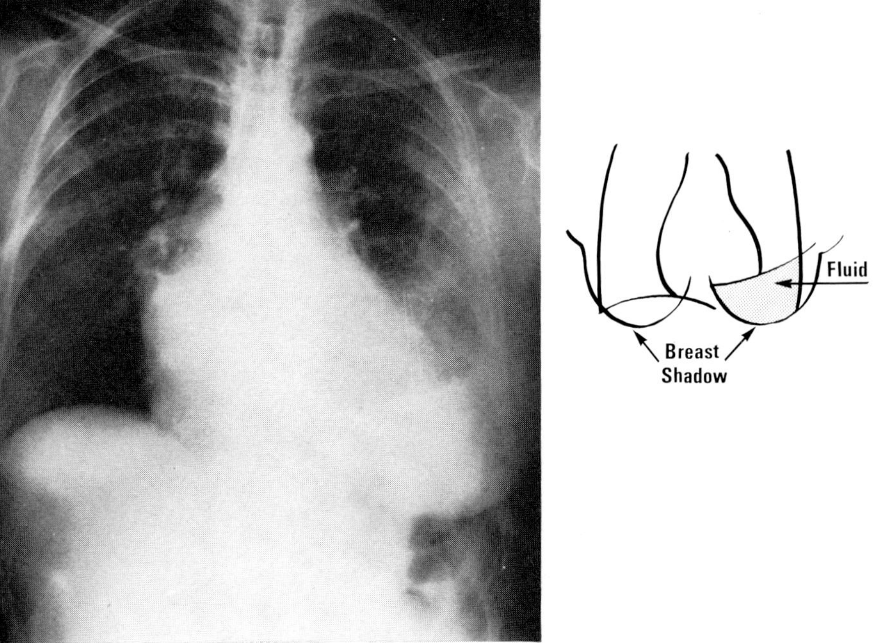

FIG. 36. Haemothorax. The X-ray shows an opacity filling the left lower pleural space. (Aspiration removed 800 ml. of blood in this case.)

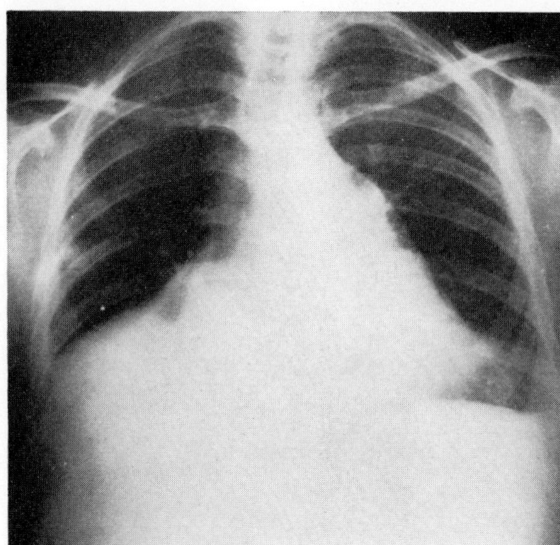

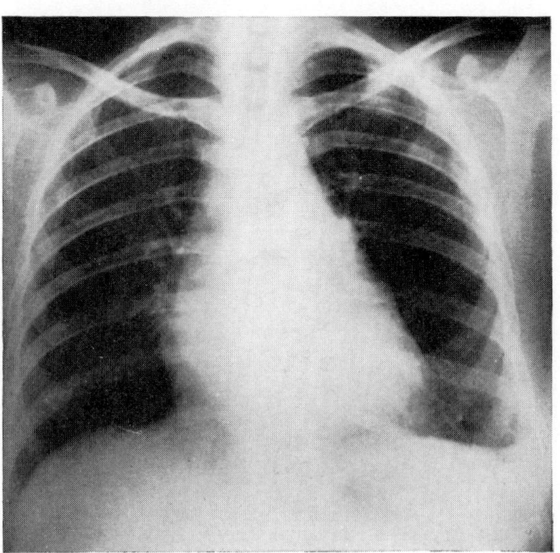

FIG. 37. Atelectasis. The upper X-ray shows absorption collapse of the lower lobe of the right lung. Energetic physiotherapy produced a plug of mucus and the lower X-ray shows re-expansion of the lung.

are impalpable and the usual sequelae of arterial blockage follow: pallor, coldness, loss of function and paraesthesiae. Embolectomy should be performed as soon as possible (p. 141).

Renal tubular necrosis

This is a complication of hypotension, particularly if it is accompanied by hypovolaemia. It can also be produced by vasopressor drugs in an ill patient whose cardiac output is low. Hypotension produces a severe vasoconstriction of the peripheral vessels in an attempt to maintain blood pressure and the severe reduction in kidney blood flow results in necrosis of the epithelium lining the renal tubules. The secretion of urine is reduced or abolished and the blood urea and blood potassium levels rise progressively. The rising blood urea causes drowsiness and eventually coma, and the high blood potassium depresses heart rate and contractility and can lead to cardiac arrest.

It is easier to prevent renal tubular damage than to treat it. If hypotension occurs during or after operation, it is routine practice to give mannitol or frusemide intravenously because these agents increase renal blood flow and urine secretion and so lessen the incidence of progressive renal damage.

If renal damage should develop in spite of these precautions, measures must be taken to reduce the formation of urea in the body and to promote excretion of urea. Dietary protein breaks down to urea in the body and a low protein, high carbohydrate diet should be given. Intravenous fluids should contain a high concentration of fructose or glucose which supply calories and reduce the breakdown of the patient's body tissues which results in urea production; 20 per cent fructose can be given into a peripheral vein but glucose is more irritant and 20 per cent glucose should be given by caval drip. Fluid intake must be restricted according to the daily urine excretion so as to avoid overhydration but, if the kidney shows a response to intravenous frusemide, this drug should be given in sufficient dosage (up to 2 g. daily) to promote a profuse diuresis. This produces a large volume of urine low in urea concentration and a diuresis of up to 6 litres urine daily may be achieved if the renal damage is not total. This large daily output may achieve sufficient excretion of urea in the urine to avert crisis levels (300 to 400 mg./100 ml. blood) and avoid the need for dialysis with the artificial kidney. When large volumes of urine are being excreted, sodium and potassium depletion are likely to occur and careful control of electrolytes is essential.

The kidney will usually recover from tubular necrosis and the rate of recovery depends on the extent of the damage to the tubular endothelium. The time required for recovery varies from 10 to 30 days and, during this time, careful assessment of blood urea and electrolytes is essential. If the blood urea and potassium levels continue to rise in spite of treatment, peritoneal or haemo-dialysis will be required. These two methods of dialysis are undertaken when the blood urea rises to 300 mg./100 ml. or higher and repeated dialysis may be required to maintain the urea at safe levels.

The fatality rate in patients developing tubular necrosis is high and the best way of avoiding it is to give mannitol and/or frusemide in the first few post-operative days so as to maintain a daily urine output of more than 1 litre.

Bacterial infection

Patients are very prone to infection after major cardiac surgery. Their defensive mechanisms are impaired by a reduced peripheral circulation, venous congestion, and the replacement of large volumes of stored blood. Bacteria can enter the blood stream via the intravascular cannulae and sampling taps; the lungs via the endotracheal tube or bronchial suction catheters; and the thoracic cavity and mediastinum via the chest drainage wounds. Patients may be nasal or skin carriers of pathogenic bacteria and cross infection from one patient to another or from staff to patient are significant hazards. Whenever possible, patients should be isolated.

The four common sites of post-operative infection are the wound, the respiratory tract, the urinary tract and the blood stream.

Wound infection. Signs of wound infection usually appear towards the end of the first post-operative week. The patient's temperature becomes elevated and he may complain of pain or discomfort in the wound. The skin surrounding the wound may be hot and red, the wound edges may be oedematous and thin blood-stained fluid may leak from between the stitches.

If a collection of fluid in the wound is suspected, one or more sutures should be removed and sinus forceps introduced to allow it to escape. A swab should be taken for bacteriological culture and sensitivity. A broad spectrum antibiotic such as ampicillin is given until the causal organism is identified and the appropriate antibiotic can be given.

Thoracotomy wounds are relatively long and care should be taken to confine the infection to its original site. If a single gauze dressing is used to cover the whole wound, it will act like a wick and lead the discharge from the infected area to the rest of the wound. Bacteria will colonise the other skin sutures and, within 48 hours, the entire wound could be in danger of dehiscence. The correct management is to cover the discharging area with a small absorbent dressing which is changed frequently, while the apparently unaffected length of the wound should be sealed off with a preparation such as Noxyflex Spray-band or Nobecutane.

Respiratory infections. These are liable to occur in patients unable or unwilling to cough effectively in the early post-operative period. Retention of secretions and atelectasis favour the onset of infection and the incidence of respiratory complications can be greatly reduced by energetic physiotherapy and by encouraging coughing.

There is a special risk in patients who require prolonged endotracheal intubation or tracheostomy. These patients cannot cough and they depend on repeated bronchial suction to keep the airway clear and avoid infection. Certain measures can be taken to facilitate the expectoration of sputum. (1) The patient should have an adequate fluid intake because dehydration results in increased viscosity of the bronchial secretions and renders them more difficult to cough up. (2) Oxygen therapy should be humified, because oxygen from the pipeline is dry, and large volumes cause drying of the main bronchi and upper respiratory tract. (3) Analgesic drugs should be used intelligently. Too much will put the patient to sleep and he will not cough; too little will leave him in pain and he cannot cough. The correct dosage is found by trial and error and this should relieve his pain without making him too drowsy to cooperate.

If infection becomes established, an antibiotic must be given and the choice of drug is dictated by the organisms cultured from the sputum.

Urinary tract infections. A complication of catheterisation of the bladder, urinary tract infections respond quickly to treatment when the catheter has been removed. They seldom retard the patient's convalescence to a significant degree, but they must be treated adequately when they occur so as to avoid the risk of leaving the patient with a sub-clinical bladder infection which is liable to recur.

Blood stream infection. Fortunately, this is a rare occurrence. When a patient has an intra-cardiac patch or artificial valve, infection becomes a disastrous complication and often leads to the death of the patient. The bacteria which enter the blood stream lodge in the plastic fabric of the patch or the valve and set up an endocarditis. This is exceedingly difficult or impossible to eradicate and the infection prevents incorporation of the patch or prosthetic valve. Recurrence of a shunt or a leak around the valve will result.

The symptoms and signs of blood stream infection are a high temperature perhaps with rigors, enlargement of the spleen, 'splinter' haemorrhages in the nail beds, haematuria, oliguria, and occasionally anuria. It is a good policy to take daily blood samples for culture during the first few days after open-heart surgery so that invasion of the blood stream by bacteria may be detected as early as possible. The organism can then be identified and its antibiotic sensitivity ascertained.

Treatment consists in giving massive doses of the appropriate antibiotic by continuous intravenous drip for a prolonged period, but the response to treatment is regrettably poor.

CHAPTER 10

Investigation of Peripheral Vascular Disease

Arteriography

This is the most important method of investigation in peripheral vascular disease. The first angiogram was performed in 1923, but the early radio-opaque drugs were irritant and this necessitated operative exposure of vessels under general anaesthesia. R. dos Santos pioneered translumbar aortography in 1929 but progress was slow until 1950 when the modern organic iodine contrast media were developed. These give excellent contrast on film and are only mildly irritant and percutaneous techniques of arteriography were developed soon after they became available. The demonstration of segmental arterial lesions which was now possible soon stimulated surgeons to undertake arterial reconstruction.

Arteriography is essential for the accurate assessment of the nature and extent of arterial disease. It provides confirmation of the diagnosis, gives a graphic illustration of the site and extent of the lesion, reveals the state of the vessel above and below the lesion and indicates the pattern of the collateral circulation. Incipient and previously unsuspected lesions are demonstrated and the accurate information essential to the selection of patients for surgery is made available.

The technique employed varies according to the part of the arterial system to be X-rayed and it is described accordingly as, for example, carotid arteriography, aortography, femoral arteriography.

Percutaneous arteriography. This is used for carotid, subclavian, brachial and femoral arteriography. It is performed by introducing a flexible plastic cannula (Fig. 38) into the artery proximal to the lesion. A suitable site is chosen where the artery is readily accessible, a skin wheal is raised with 1 per cent Lignocaine (plain) and local anaesthetic is injected into the subcutaneous tissues and around the artery. A small nick is made in the skin with a scalpel to permit easy entry of the cannula. A sharp steel needle and stillette fit snugly inside the Teflon cannula which is introduced through the skin until it enters the artery. The needle and stillette are withdrawn and blood jets from the end of the cannula. This is connected to dye filled tubing leading from a syringe filled with the volume of dye to be injected. Injection may be performed by emptying the syringe manually or the radiologist may actuate a compressed air

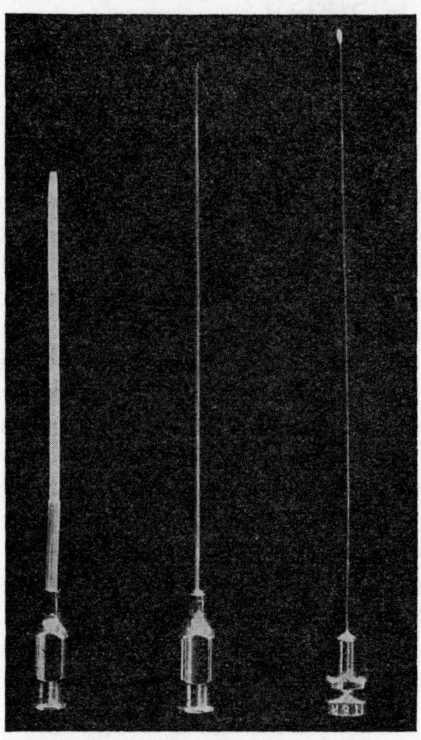

FIG. 38. Teflon cannula for percutaneous arteriography. On the left is the cannula, and, on the right, a needle and stillette which fit snugly inside the cannula.

pump which empties the syringe at a predetermined pressure. Dye is introduced rapidly and forcibly into the artery and, depending on circumstances, a single film or multiple films in an automatic cassette changer are exposed.

Percutaneous femoral catheterisation. This method was introduced by Seldinger (p. 19) in 1953. A long radio-opaque catheter is introduced into the femoral artery in the groin and passed up under the visual control of an image intensifier into the abdominal aorta —aortography, or up to the aortic arch—arch aortography. In certain circumstances, a catheter with a bend at the tip is introduced into a specific artery and a bolus of dye is injected directly into that vessel—selective visceral arteriography.

Translumbar aortography. Used in the investigation of occlusions of the aorta and its branches, translumbar aortography is necessary when the Seldinger catheter cannot be passed up the iliac arteries. It is performed under general anaesthesia with the patient in the prone position. The skin below the left 12th rib and lateral to the spinal muscles is pierced with a scalpel and a long arterial cannula is directed forwards and medially until it meets the bony resistance of the vertebral column. The cannula is partly withdrawn and directed more anteriorly to enter the aorta. It is attached to the prefilled tubing and syringe and 30 ml. dye is injected forcibly by a compressed air pump. A series of films is exposed at pre-set intervals by the automatic cassette changer.

When films of the legs are also required, a moving table top is set in motion and the patient is carried headwards over the cassette changer so that films can be taken of the femoral, popliteal and tibial arteries while the dye is being carried down the legs by the flow of blood.

COMPLICATIONS

Complications are rare and arteriography is relatively safe in fit patients. Sometimes, however, films are unsatisfactory due to technical errors, extravasation of dye, or poor timing, and the investigation has to be repeated.

Haemorrhage is rarely serious although occasionally a haematoma may occur. Needless to say, arteriography must never be undertaken while the patient is on anti-coagulants.

Iodism and allergic reactions to the dye are rare but it has been estimated that fatal reactions may occur in 1:120,000 injections. A test dose of 1 ml. dye is injected intravenously prior to arteriography in order to detect the possibility of allergy.

Renal and spinal cord damage may occur, especially in translumbar aortography, if a large volume of dye is injected directly into a renal or lumbar artery. In most cases, the damage is temporary and reversible but renal infarct, tubular necrosis or paraplegia can occur.

Arterial injury may occur if the intima or an atherosclerotic plaque is stripped up by the forcible dye injection or dislodged by the Seldinger catheter. Urgent operation may be necessary to explore and repair the damaged artery.

Skin temperature measurement

When thermocouples are attached to the skin a minute electric current is generated. This current is proportional to the skin temperature and can be measured on a galvanometer. The temperature of the skin depends primarily on the blood flow through it and cutaneous vasodilation induced by warming raises the skin temperature. When the main artery to the limb is blocked, the consequent reduction in blood flow keeps the skin cooler than in a normal limb despite full cutaneous vasodilation.

In the vasodilation test, thermocouples are attached to both great toes. The rate and extent of temperature increase in the toes is governed by the site and extent of the arterial occlusion and the efficiency of the collateral circulation. This test gives a measure of the efficiency of the collateral circulation and is a guide, within certain limitations, to the improvement in skin circulation attainable after sympathectomy.

The investigation is undertaken in a room thermostatically controlled at 21°C (70°F). Thermocouples are attached to both great toes and readings are taken at five minute intervals. When three readings have given a base line (usually about 18° to 20°C) the arms are immersed in water whose temperature is 49°C (120°F). Where there is no occlusion, a normal S-shaped curve is obtained (Fig. 39) with the rise commencing within 10 minutes of immersion and levelling off around 30°C (86°F). When occlusion is present, the rise is delayed and the level eventually reached is usually less than normal. In general, the more distal the lesion the flatter the curve (Fig. 39).

Oscillometry

The oscillometer is an instrument which measures arterial pulsation. A double cuff similar to that of a sphygmomanometer is placed around the thigh or calf and the proximal cuff is inflated. Arterial pulsation transmitted to the lower cuff is recorded by a needle oscillating on a gauge and readings are taken with different pressures in the proximal cuff so as to determine the maximum oscillation of the needle.

The range of oscillation of the needle is reduced in atherosclerosis and is minimal or absent when the main artery is occluded. However, this information has only a limited value in supporting the findings made on clinical examination.

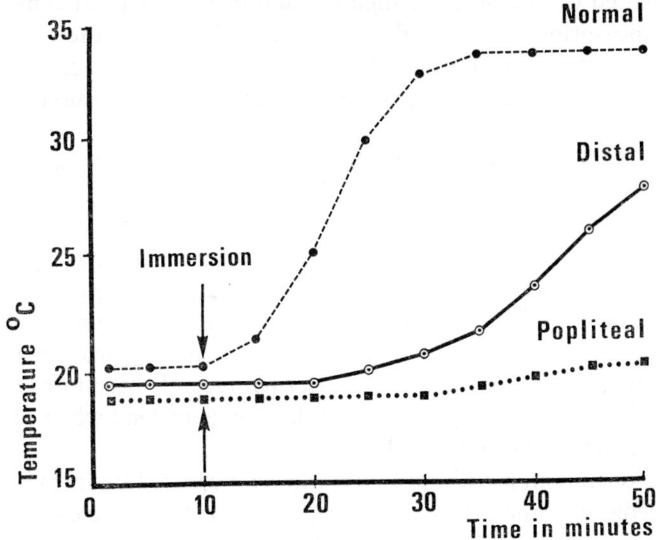

FIG. 39. Vasodilation test, illustrating three types of curve commonly obtained. The 'distal' type of curve is obtained with most femoro-popliteal occlusions and the 'popliteal' curve with popliteal occlusions where the collateral circulation is poor.

Ergometry

The claudication distance (p. 111) of a patient varies according to the speed of walking and the inclination of the ground. Various walking machines are available with a moving platform on which the patient stands, and, when it is set in motion, he has to walk in order to maintain his position. Unfortunately, the energy expended by the calf muscles on this machine is different from that of normal walking and the method has a limited use in measuring the patient's disability.

A simpler method is the two-step test where the patient walks up two steps then down again and continues doing so at a set speed until calf pain is produced.

Plethysmography

If venous return from a digit or limb is prevented by a venous tourniquet, blood continues to flow through the arteries and the tissues beyond the tourniquet increase in volume. This can be measured by encasing the digit or limb in a water filled container and measuring the rate of displacement of the water. Alternatively, a strain-gauge can be placed round the part and the changes in strain which occur with increased volume can be measured.

There are numerous other methods of investigation available, but most of these are used in research rather than in routine clinical work.

The *electrical conductivity of the skin* can be used as an index of sympathetic activity. *Radioactive isotopes* can be injected into the leg muscles and the rate of clearance measured. *Oxygen tension* in leg muscles can be recorded by special electrodes introduced into the muscle. An *ultrasonic flow detector* has recently been introduced and this instrument gives an audible change of tone when placed over a stenosed or occluded artery.

At operation, *arterial pressures* can be measured by introducing a needle into the artery and the gradient between proximal and distal pressures can be measured, e.g., in renal artery stenosis. *Blood flow measurement* can also be done by placing an electro-magnetic flowmeter probe around the exposed artery.

CHAPTER 11

Atherosclerosis

This is a condition of middle age and later life, which produces changes in the arterial wall and leads to such diverse conditions as coronary and cerebral thrombosis, gangrene of the extremities, and aneurysms.

In this disease, lipids (particles of fat) are deposited in the arterial wall. Although the disease is normally regarded as one in which the principal changes occur in the intima (Fig. 40) important changes affect all layers of the artery.

During life, the structure of an artery undergoes change. In early years, a healthy artery develops cushion-like thickenings at the major branches in response to the stress of arterial pulsation. With increasing age, lipids are deposited in the deeper layers of the intima and these deposits increase in size to form atherosclerotic plaques. At the same time, there is disruption of the internal elastic lamina, progressive replacement of the muscle in the media by fibrous tissue, and a variable amount of fibrosis in and around the outer adventitial coat of the artery. As the plaque increases in size, haemorrhage may occur into it leading to further production of lipids, and calcium salts may be deposited in the plaques or in the medial coat. When calcified, the plaque may ulcerate through the endothelial lining and platelets are deposited on the surface to form platelet thrombus. This can become detached and plug a distal artery, or slowly enlarge in situ until it blocks the artery.

There are many theories put forward to explain the accumulation of lipids in atherosclerosis. In general, it can be said that there are a number of general factors governing the onset and severity of the disease in any individual, and there is a second set of mechanical factors which decide the localisation of plaques in different parts of the arterial system of that individual.

General factors

Atherosclerosis is a disease of civilised races and this may be related to *racial inheritance* or to *diet*. Some individuals have a congenitally high level of fat (*hyperlipidaemia*) or cholesterol (*hypercholesterolaemia*) in the blood and are thus subject to the disease.

Others have a high dietary intake of fat and excess of saturated fats in the diet has been implicated as a predisposing cause. On the other hand, excessive carbohydrate consumption has also been blamed, and the high incidence of coronary disease in Glasgow is thought to be related to the softness of the water supply. The exact role of dietary factors is uncertain and, although a diet of unsaturated (mainly vegetable) fats is frequently advocated, there is insufficient evidence as yet to say that any one type of diet is beneficial in prevention of the disease.

Men are about six times more liable to atherosclerotic vascular disease than women and there is good experimental evidence to indicate that oestrogens exert a protective effect against the development of atheroma, although oestrogens are ineffective as a form of treatment once the disease has developed.

Diabetes mellitus is associated with hypercholesterolaemia and diabetic patients, including women, have a high incidence of atherosclerosis which tends to develop at an earlier age than otherwise.

Localising factors

Intimal thickening of a minor degree may be a physiological reaction to mechanical stress but lipid deposition is pathological and results in the formation of atherosclerotic plaques (Fig. 41).

The commonest site of plaque formation in the peripheral arteries is in the thigh—in the adductor canal and at the adductor opening where the femoral artery passes through the tendon of the adductor magnus muscle to reach the popliteal fossa behind the knee and become the popliteal artery (Fig. 42). In this region, the mechanical stress produced by arterial pulsation against a fixed unyielding tendon, the presence of several large arterial branches, and the crossing of the artery by numerous small veins may all play a part in causing the mechanical stress which produces the arterial lesion.

Plaques also tend to form at the sites of origin of branches, e.g., the aortic, common iliac, popliteal, carotid bifurcations, etc. They also tend to form in the proximal few centimetres of large vessels, e.g., coronary, superior mesenteric. Plaques are common in the larger arteries where mechanical stress is greatest, and are usually few or absent in the smaller vessels.

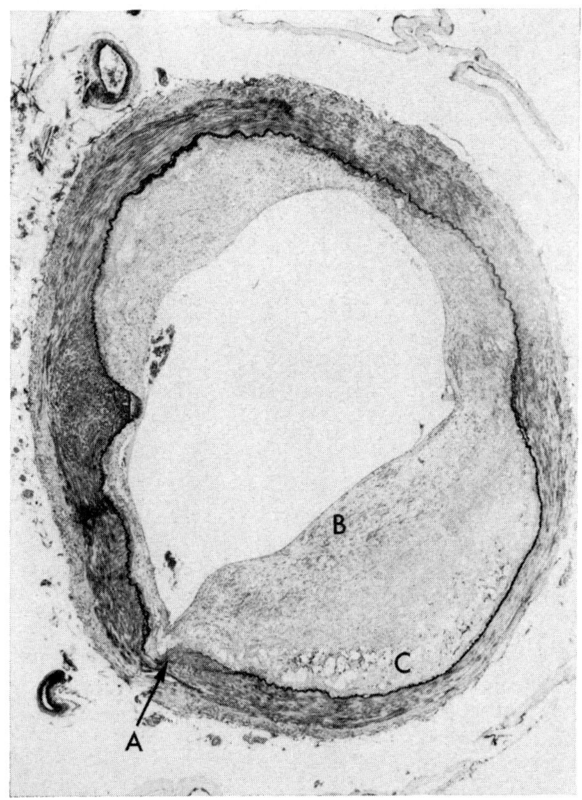

FIG. 40. Transverse section of atheromatous artery. The internal elastic lamina is attenuated and disrupted (A), the intima is grossly thickened (B), and lipids are deposited in the deeper layers of the intima (C).

To face page 100

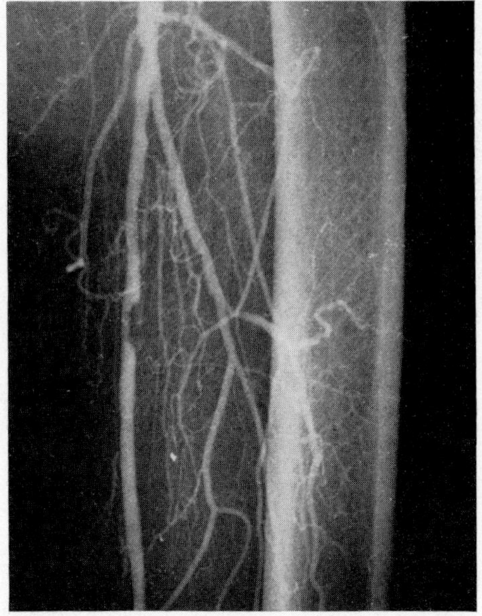

FIG. 41. Femoral arteriogram showing a large atheromatous plaque in the upper part of the superficial femoral artery. The deep femoral artery inclines towards the femur and gives rise to numerous collateral branches.

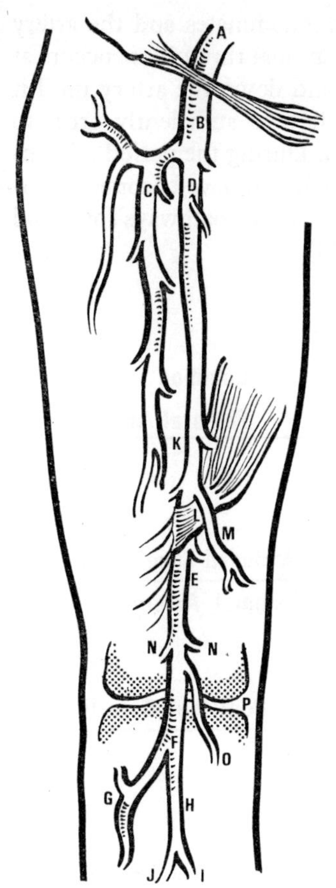

FIG. 42. The femoral and popliteal arteries and their branches. A external iliac artery, B common femoral artery, C deep femoral artery, D superficial femoral artery, E popliteal artery, F popliteal bifurcation, G anterior tibial artery, H posterior tibial stem, I posterior tibial artery, J peroneal artery, K adductor canal, L adductor tendon, M descending genicular artery, N genicular arteries, O sural artery, P knee joint.

Arterial changes

The diameter of the arterial lumen tends to be reduced by *intimal thickening and plaque formation* and, in the course of time, thrombosis occurs at the narrowed area and blocks the artery. On the other hand, disruption of the elastic lamina and *fibrosis of the media* weaken the arterial wall and the force of arterial pressure tends to cause dilatation and aneurysm formation. A third relatively minor feature is *periarterial fibrosis* which tends to constrict the artery but this is rarely severe enough to cause trouble. The results of atherosclerosis depend on which of these features is most prominent.

In most cases, intimal thickening predominates and the artery becomes progressively narrowed. When final thrombosis occurs at any point, the thrombus spreads up and down the artery until it meets a side-channel whose rate of flow is sufficiently great to prevent further extension of thrombus. During the period of stenosis, the branches above and below the lesion have become gradually larger in size so as to establish alternative pathways for blood flow—the *collateral circulation* (Fig. 43).

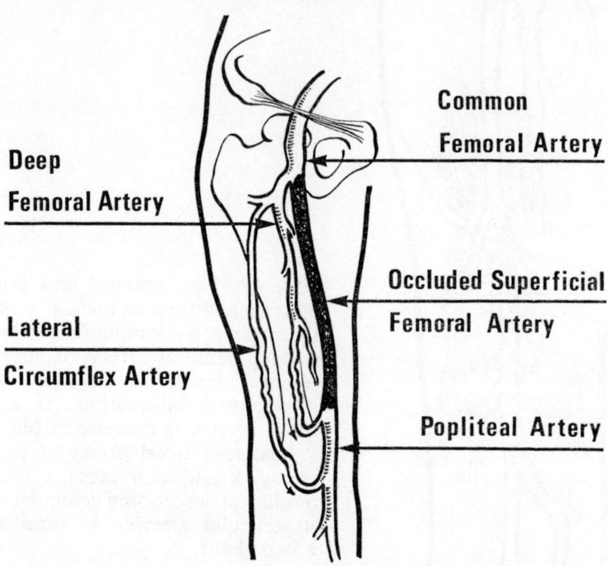

FIG. 43. Collateral circulation. When the superficial femoral artery is occluded, the deep femoral artery forms anastomotic communications with the branches of the popliteal artery so as to convey blood to the distal parts of the limb.

When the artery becomes occluded these enlarged branches carry blood through the side channels to the tissues below the occlusion. The normal direction of blood flow is reversed in the collateral branches which carry blood back into the distal main artery. The clinical effects of this thrombosis depend on the efficiency of the collateral circulation which itself depends on such factors as the age of the patient, and the site and extent of the arterial occlusion.

In a minority of cases, weakening of the arterial wall is the principal feature and arterial dilatation occurs. Progressive dilatation of one part of the arterial system leads to the formation of an *aneurysm* which enlarges steadily until the tissues are unable to contain it. Rupture of the wall of the aneurysm leads to profuse bleeding which is usually fatal. While the aneurysm is enlarging, thrombus is being laid down on the inner lining of the sac and, at any time, this process may predominate and lead to thrombosis of the aneurysm.

CHAPTER 12

Aneurysms

An aneurysm is a blood-containing sac connected with an artery. It may be described as a *true* aneurysm, a swelling of the arterial wall itself, or as a *false* aneurysm, a cavity in the soft tissues which connects with an artery (Fig. 44). True aneurysms may be *fusiform*,

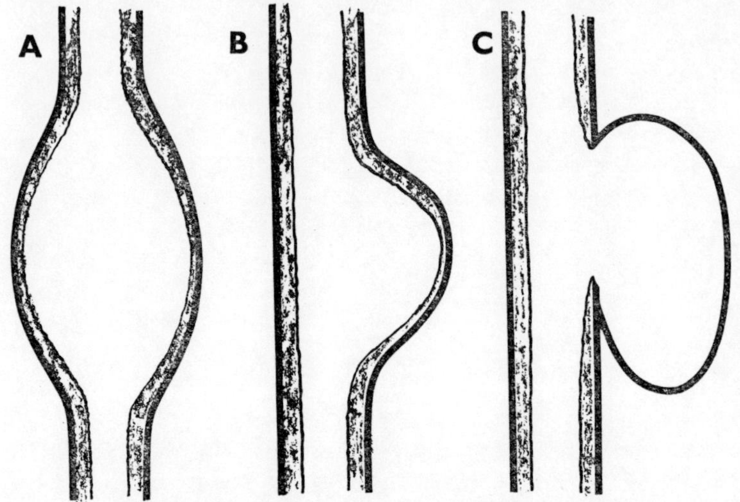

FIG. 44. Aneurysms. A Fusiform. B Saccular. C False.

a symmetrical dilatation of the arterial wall, or *saccular*, where one wall of the artery dilates and forms a sac connected to the artery by a wide mouth.

Aneurysms may result from different causes. They may be *congenital* in origin as, for example, in the intracranial aneurysms which form in the circle of Willis at congenitally weak portions of the arterial wall and give rise to intracranial haemorrhage in early adult life. They may be *traumatic* in origin where the artery is punctured by a sharp instrument and the resultant haematoma remains in communication with the artery and gradually forms a false aneurysm. They may be *infective* in origin due to weakening of the vessel wall produced by syphilitic arteritis or by infection from infected emboli (p. 140). They may be caused by *disease* such as atherosclerosis which produces weakness of the arterial wall.

Most of the aneurysms dealt with by the cardio-vascular surgeon are due to atherosclerosis and the commonest site at which aneurysms develop is in the abdominal aorta between the renal arteries and the aortic bifurcation—*abdominal aneurysm* (Fig. 45). The diseased aorta becomes elongated and tortuous and this, together with the dilatation, often results in the aneurysm lying mainly to one side of the midline, usually the left. Calcium is deposited in the wall of the aneurysm and layers of thrombus are deposited on the inner wall of the sac although a central channel remains in which the flow of blood is maintained. Increasing dilatation leads to rupture of the bulging arterial wall and the patient will die if surgery is delayed. Occasionally thrombus formation predominates over dilatation and thrombosis results.

Dilatation of the common iliac arteries frequently accompanies aneurysm of the abdominal aorta and aneurysms occur also in the internal iliac, femoral and popliteal arteries. Aneurysms of the aortic arch, the thoracic aorta and the visceral arteries (e.g., renal, splenic, mesenteric) are not uncommon.

Clinical features

Because atherosclerosis is a degenerative process, most aneurysms occur in patients over 60 years of age and they are commoner in men than women. Some may have had a previous coronary artery thrombosis or a 'shock' due to a cerebro-vascular incident. Aneurysms of the abdomen, neck or limbs can be recognised as tense swellings which pulsate with each heart beat and seem to expand as they do so, i.e., they show 'expansile pulsation'. They cause pain when their gradual expansion produces pressure on neighbouring structures or when a leak or rupture occurs.

Aneurysms present in four ways:

1. As a pulsating lump, they may be noticed by the patient or found by the doctor during routine examination. At this stage they are usually symptomless.

2. Pressure on neighbouring organs may give rise to mild symptoms of abdominal discomfort, nausea and flatulence. Erosion of the vertebral column (either thoracic or lumbar) can give rise to pain in the back.

3. An episode of more severe pain of sudden onset due to a leak from the aneurysm.

4. Acute pain, collapse, rapid thready pulse, and low blood pressure due to rupture of the aneurysm and severe blood loss.

Treatment

The only worth-while treatment of aneurysm is replacement of the dilated portion of artery by a Dacron or Teflon graft (Fig. 46). This is not a formidable operation when the patient is fit, and the operative mortality is reasonably low (less than 10 per cent) when operation is undertaken before the stage of rupture. When rupture has occurred, operation is hazardous and carries a mortality rate of 50 to 75 per cent, but without operation rupture is almost invariably fatal.

As the time which elapses between diagnosis of an average sized aneurysm and death from rupture is approximately one year, operation should be advised in all patients who are reasonably fit or in those whose normal life expectancy can be regarded as more than one year.

PRE-OPERATIVE

The preparation of a patient with an unruptured aneurysm is the same as for aorto-iliac operations (Chap. 23).

When the aneurysm has ruptured and the patient is still alive on admission to hospital, the surgeon must decide whether operation is possible or not. If the patient was in good health prior to the onset of rupture, it is usually worth while to attempt emergency resection and grafting. An intravenous plasma drip is set up, 10 or more pints of blood are cross-matched by emergency methods, and operation is commenced as soon as blood is available.

OPERATION

Anaesthesia is rapidly induced but muscle relaxants are not given until the surgeon has completed his incision, because relaxation of the abdominal muscles lowers the intra-abdominal pressure and can lead to severe haemorrhage before the surgeon is in a position to control the aorta above the aneurysm.

When the abdomen is opened, the diagnosis is usually obvious because of the severe retroperitoneal bleeding which is present. Bowel is displaced to the right, the posterior parietal peritoneum is incised above the aneurysm, and the aorta below the renal arteries is rapidly dissected free from surrounding tissue and a large De

Bakey clamp is applied (Fig. 47). When the aorta has been clamped, bleeding is controlled and the anaesthetist is able to transfuse sufficient blood to restore normal blood pressure.

Further procedure does not need to be hurried and the rest of the operation is performed in the same way as an elective operation for aneurysm.

The common iliac arteries are now examined. If they are relatively normal in size, a large diameter single tubular graft can be sutured to the aortic bifurcation and the common iliac arteries can be clamped just below the aortic bifurcation. If the common iliac arteries are dilated, a bifurcation graft will be required and the surgeon has to decide where the lower anastomosis will be. He can perform an end-to-end anastomosis between the graft and common iliac artery or he can suture the end of the graft to the side of the common iliac, external iliac or common femoral artery, i.e., an end-to-side anastomosis. When this has been decided, clamps are placed below the intended lower anastomosis.

The inferior mesenteric artery is divided between ligatures as it emerges from the left side of the dilated aorta and a longitudinal incision is made into the sac. The layers of thrombus are removed together with as much of the intima as possible. The lumbar arteries can now be seen bleeding back into the sac and they are underrun with a silk suture to stop bleeding.

The graft is cut to the desired length and the upper end is sutured to the aorta at the upper end of the sac with a continuous 3/O or 4/O nonabsorbable suture. The lower anastomosis is performed and the cut edges of the sac are sutured together in front of the graft so as to encase it within the aneurysmal sac. The peritoneum and wound are now closed.

POST-OPERATIVE

The post-operative management is similar to that for aorto-iliac operations (p. 148). Most of these patients are elderly and unfit and cardio-respiratory problems are numerous during recovery. The prolonged hypotension which occurs after rupture may produce renal tubular necrosis (p. 89) and management of urinary function in these patients is very important.

DISSECTING ANEURYSM

This is a special type of aneurysm which is an uncommon cause of sudden death. If an atherosclerotic area of the aorta becomes necrotic, the flow of blood may raise a flap of intima which becomes progressively stripped up as blood passes down in the wall of the artery. This dissection usually commences in the region of the aortic arch but it may begin lower down. A false channel is formed between the inner and outer coats of the artery and, if this ruptures outwards, the patient will die from haemorrhage into the thorax or abdomen. If the blood flowing down the false channel ruptures back into the lumen of the artery, the situation may remain stable long enough to give the surgeon time to plan and undertake operation.

The pressure of the blood flowing in the false channel compresses or occludes the normal channel and blood flow into the legs is obstructed if the dissection extends down to or beyond the aortic bifurcation. The renal arteries may be compressed or short-circuited by the dissection and irreversible kidney damage may be caused by inadequate renal blood flow. If the patient becomes anuric, operation is unlikely to be of value.

Clinically, the patient develops severe chest or abdominal pain with severe back pain, hypotension and a rapid pulse. Weakness of the legs and alteration in the volume of the femoral pulses are important diagnostic features of the condition.

Operation can be performed in one of two ways. An attempt can be made to repair the aorta at the site of the original dissection or the surgeon can enlarge the 'window' where the false channel has ruptured back into the lumen. With either method, the mortality of operation is high but it is the only chance for survival of the patient.

CHAPTER 13

Arterial Occlusion in the Lower Limb

ATHEROSCLEROSIS

The commonest cause of ischaemia in the lower limb is atherosclerosis and the flow of blood into the leg can be reduced by any lesion which causes stenosis or occlusion of the aorta or of a major artery in the leg. The intimal thickening caused by atherosclerosis affects most of the large arteries although the deep femoral artery, the peroneal artery, and the smaller arteries tend to remain relatively free from disease. Atherosclerosis can be diagnosed from the arteriogram which shows irregularity of outline and a reduction in vessel diameter.

PATTERN OF ARTERIAL LESIONS

As lipids are deposited in increasing amounts, atherosclerotic plaques develop at certain sites. In the aorto-iliac segment, plaque formation is commonest at the aortic bifurcation, in the middle of the common iliac artery and at the common iliac bifurcation. In the femoro-popliteal segment, 70 per cent of lesions occur at the adductor opening or in the adductor canal, and most of the remainder affect the popliteal artery above the level of the knee joint or at the popliteal bifurcation. The common femoral artery often shows plaque formation but occlusion is uncommon because of the large volume of blood flowing into the branches of the deep femoral artery.

There is a great variety in the types of lesion produced and a full discussion of these is beyond the scope of this book. The commonest lesion originates at the adductor region and causes stenosis or occlusion of the superficial femoral artery at this site. As the lesion progresses, the branches of the femoral and popliteal arteries enlarge to form the collateral circulation. When occlusion occurs, thrombosis extends up and down as far as the nearest branches although small branches may be overwhelmed by the spreading thrombus, and the length of the occlusion depends on the size and site of origin of these branches.

The principal collateral vessel in the thigh is the deep femoral artery (Fig. 43) and the severity of ischaemia depends to a large extent on the level to which the occlusion extends distally, i.e., an occlusion affecting a large part of the popliteal artery causes a more severe reduction in blood flow than an occlusion of the superficial femoral artery alone because fewer and smaller branches of the profunda are available to anastomose with the branches of the popliteal artery. Proximal extension of the adductor occlusion has little effect on symptoms because the deep femoral collateral flow to the main artery below the occlusion is not affected. On the other hand, distal extension of an adductor occlusion reduces the number of re-entrant collaterals and increases the severity of the ischaemia.

In general, the more proximal an occlusion is situated the better is the collateral flow because the branches are larger and more numerous. Aortic and iliac occlusions develop excellent collaterals whereas popliteal and tibial occlusions do not. Double occlusions (e.g. the combination of a common iliac and a femoro-popliteal occlusion) can produce severe ischaemia. Bilateral disease is common and 70 per cent of patients with a femoro-popliteal occlusion have stenosis or occlusion in the other leg. The incidence of tibial occlusion associated with femoro-popliteal occlusion is high—approximately 50 per cent. Sometimes, the anterior and posterior tibial arteries are both occluded leaving the peroneal artery as the only supply of blood to the foot. This lesion is called 'peroneal leg' and it occurs in 10 per cent of claudicating patients and in almost 40 per cent of legs amputated for gangrene.

RESULTS OF ARTERIAL OCCLUSION

When a leg artery becomes narrowed or blocked, blood flow to the tissue beyond the lesion is reduced and either muscle or skin or both may show signs of this diminished circulation.

When the deficiency is not too severe, the muscles distal to the occlusion do not receive sufficient blood flow to permit prolonged repeated contraction. As they work, the waste products of muscle metabolism accumulate until the sensory nerve endings are stimulated and pain is produced. When the muscle stops contracting, the waste products are gradually metabolised by the continuing supply of oxygen and the muscle returns to a more normal and healthy state. Further exercise provokes the cycle once again. With a limited circulation, therefore, there is a limit to the amount of work a muscle can do before pain makes the patient stop walking.

This type of pain is called *exercise pain.* When only one leg is affected, the patient often limps so as to reduce the amount of work done by that leg and exercise pain is usually called *intermittent claudication* (Latin: claudicare: to limp).

When the circulatory deficiency is severe, the skin and other tissues may not receive sufficient blood to nourish them and *gangrene* develops where the arterial deficiency is most severe, namely, in the toes (Fig. 48). When the circulation to the toes is reduced gradually, the tissues shrivel and become black and mummified—*dry gangrene.* If the arterial circulation is suddenly cut off, the tissues retain fluid—*moist gangrene.* This latter type occurs in embolism and diabetes mellitus and the moist tissues are vulnerable to infection which can spread rapidly.

As gangrene develops, the patient experiences pain because the sensory nerve endings in skin are stimulated by the ischaemia. This pain is unrelated to exercise and is often worse when the patient is in bed—hence it is called *ischaemic rest pain.*

SYMPTOMS

Arterial occlusion of the legs due to atherosclerosis is commoner in men than women (6:1 ratio) and almost all these patients smoke cigarettes. The largest group is aged 50 to 60 years but the disease can affect patients in their twenties and thirties.

The majority of patients present with intermittent claudication which may be unilateral or bilateral. The onset is usually insidious and only gradually does the patient become aware that he develops pain in the calf muscle when he walks a long distance. If the arterial lesion is progressive, he finds that he requires to stop after shorter and shorter distances until he can walk only 50 to 100 yards. The claudication distance varies with the speed of walking and with the inclination of the ground, the distance being severely reduced on walking uphill.

Some patients have an apparently sudden onset of symptoms following a period of bed rest due to operation or illness. The explanation is that thrombosis has taken place during inactivity and only on the resumption of normal activity does he find that he cannot walk far.

In most patients, an efficient collateral circulation develops and the claudication distance becomes stable. Only a minority deteriorate and develop gangrene.

If the circulation deteriorates, rest pain may develop without actual gangrene. When the patient goes to bed the temperature of the feet is raised by virtue of their being covered and this increased tissue temperature makes greater demands on an already inadequate circulation. The patient finds that he can obtain relief from pain by getting out of bed or by walking about because this lowers the temperature of the toes to that of the room and also adds the force of gravity to help arterial flow to the legs. Occasionally, merely elevating the head of the bed will improve the circulation sufficiently to relieve rest pain.

This stage of incipient gangrene is often associated with cold feet, numbness in the toes, or ulceration. Spontaneous relief of rest pain may occur if there is an adequate improvement in the collateral circulation but, if not, rest pain continues and signs of gangrene appear.

Gangrene may therefore occur as a sequel to claudication when there is progressive deterioration of the circulation. In many patients, however, the initial arterial thrombosis is extensive and incipient or established gangrene develops without preliminary claudication. Pain is persistent and, as it is always worst in bed, the patient sleeps with his legs hanging out of bed, spends his nights sleeping in a chair, or does not sleep at all. He becomes tired and anxious, loses weight and his general condition deteriorates.

CLINICAL SIGNS

Pulse patterns. When arterial occlusion develops, pulsation is diminished or absent in the main artery below the lesion. By careful palpation, it is possible to detect pulsation (or its absence) in the main artery at various accessible sites and to deduce the level of occlusion. This lies below the most distal normal pulse.

In the leg, the pulses examined are the femoral pulse in the groin, the popliteal pulse behind the knee, the posterior tibial pulse behind the medial malleolus, and the dorsalis pedis on top of the foot.

It is desirable to have a system by which pulses can be recorded in the case notes. This may differ in various units but a simple and satisfactory system is: $+$ = normal pulsation; $-$ = absent pulsation; $\pm$ = diminished pulsation. If the femoral, popliteal, posterior tibial and dorsalis pedis pulses are charted in a consistent order, the pulse chart of a leg can be represented as $+ + + +$. If

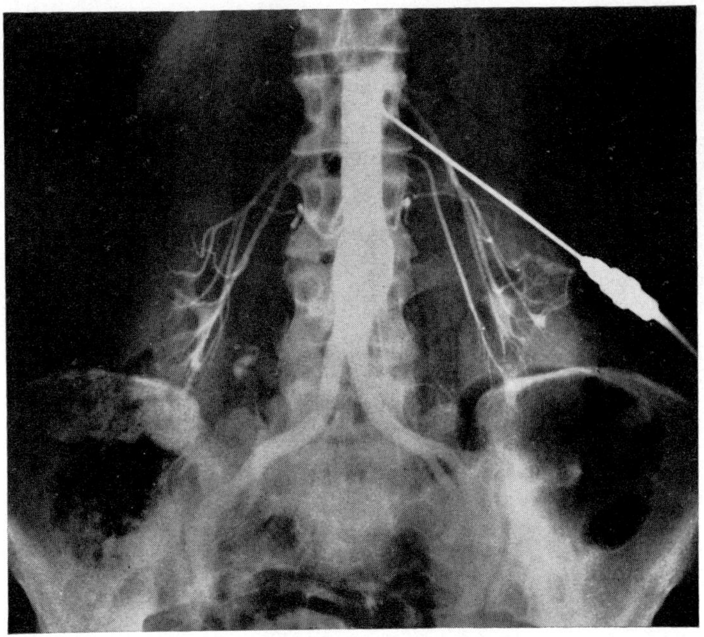

Fig. 45. Fusiform aneurysm of the abdominal aorta due to atherosclerosis in a woman of 45 years.

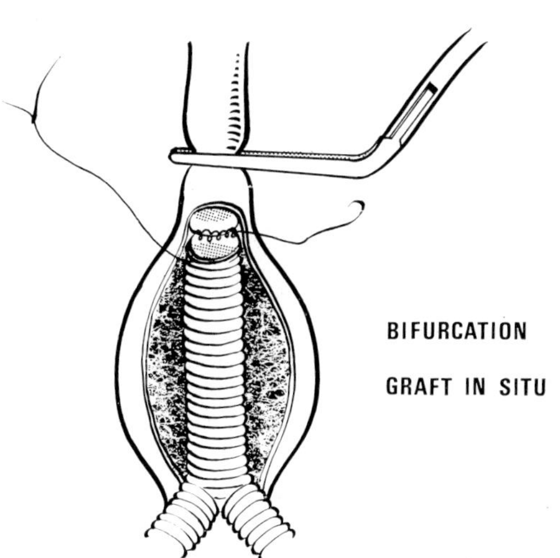

Fig. 46. Graft replacement in abdominal aneurysm. The Dacron graft is placed inside the sac of the aneurysm and sutured to the abdominal aorta at the level where the artery begins to dilate.

To face page 112

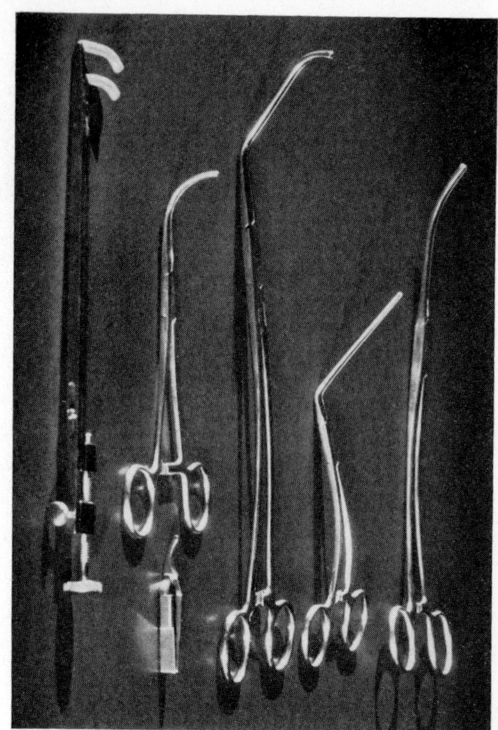

FIG. 47. Arterial clamps. Left to right: Blalock clamp, De Bakey curved clamp with bulldog clamp below, Satinsky clamp, De Bakey angled clamp, and a large De Bakey arterial clamp.

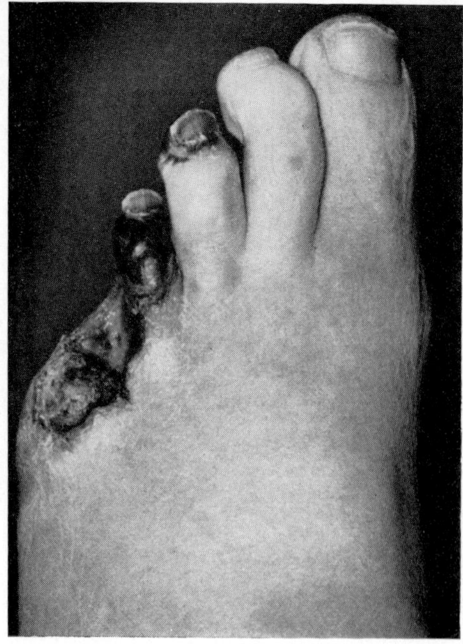

FIG. 48. Dry gangrene of the fourth toe and the tip of the third. The fifth toe has already separated.

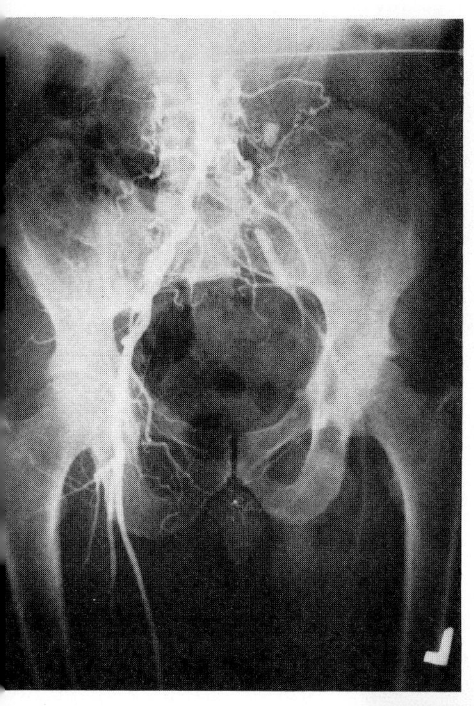

FIG. 49. Occlusion of the left common iliac artery; the dye shadow in the distal vessels on the left side is less intense because blood has to flow through the collateral circulation to reach the main artery below the occlusion.

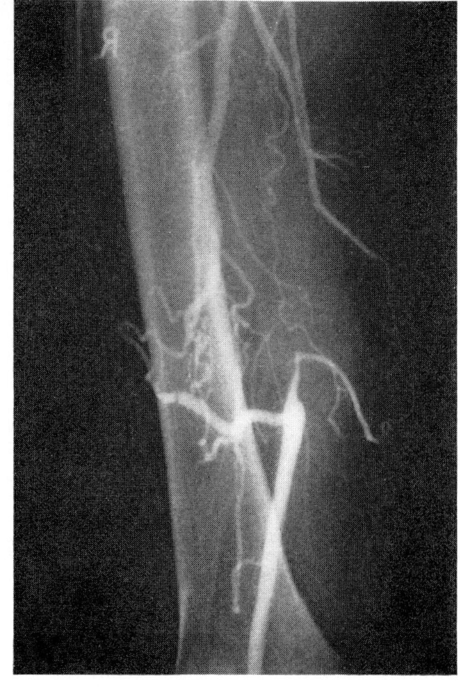

IG. 50. Occlusion of the superficial femoral artery.

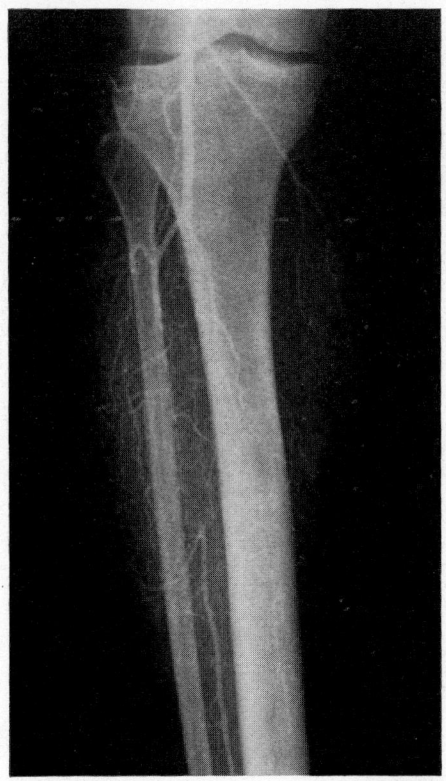

FIG. 51. Occlusion of the anter and posterior tibial arteries. T peroneal artery is reconstitu about mid-calf level.

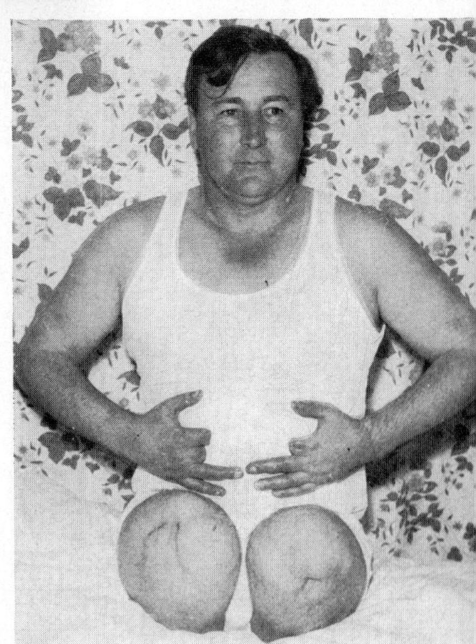

FIG. 52. Thrombo-angiitis obliterans. This has resulted in bilateral mid-thigh amputations and the loss of three fingers.

the two legs are charted together, always with the right leg charted above the left, the whole chart becomes $\genfrac{}{}{0pt}{}{++++}{++++}$.

Some common abnormal pulse patterns are as follows:

$\genfrac{}{}{0pt}{}{++++}{----}$ This indicates normal pulsation in the right leg and absent pulsation in the left leg due to a block situated above the groin—i.e., in either the common or external iliac artery (Fig. 49).

$\genfrac{}{}{0pt}{}{----}{----}$ This shows absent pulsation in both legs due to occlusion of the aorta. It could also be caused by bilateral occlusion of the external iliac or common femoral arteries but these lesions are rare. It could not be due to bilateral occlusion of the common iliac arteries because, if this should occur, thrombosis would be propagated up into the aorta and the occlusion would be aortic.

$\genfrac{}{}{0pt}{}{++++}{+---}$ This is the commonest pulse pattern of all which indicates an arterial block in the left thigh, i.e., below the level of the femoral pulse and above that of the popliteal pulse (Fig. 50).

$\genfrac{}{}{0pt}{}{++--}{++++}$ This chart shows normal pulsation in the right thigh and absence of both right ankle pulses—i.e. occlusion of the distal part of the right popliteal artery or occlusion of both tibial arteries. This pattern is common in diabetic patients (Fig. 51).

In some patients, there is a palpable *thrill* when a pulse is felt and in others an audible *bruit* can be heard with each heart beat when a stethoscope is placed over the artery. This is due to turbulent flow in the artery caused by stenosis or dilatation and is an important sign in internal carotid stenosis and in aneurysms.

COLOUR CHANGES

When arterial circulation is deficient, colour changes occur when the leg is raised or lowered. Raising the leg leads to *blanching* of the foot and the rate at which blanching develops and the height to which the leg must be raised to produce it give some measure of the deficiency in blood flow. In severe ischaemia, dangling the leg produces a red discolouration of the skin of the foot—*dependency rubor*. Again, the intensity of the colour and the rate at which it develops are indicative of the severity of the circulatory deficiency.

Sometimes in the fingers and toes *cyanosis* appears due to sluggish circulation. Under these circumstances, the tissues remove most of the oxygen from the blood and the haemoglobin of the blood changes from the bright red oxyhaemoglobin to the dark purple colour of reduced haemoglobin. This colour change is often a pre-gangrenous one.

When tissues become *white*, there is virtually no blood flow through the part. This may be seen when the artery of a limb is suddenly blocked by an embolus and blood is squeezed out of the distal vessels. It also occurs in Raynaud's phenomenon when the fingers blanch on exposure to cold.

Trophic and other changes. Muscles waste when their blood supply is inadequate and inequality in size of the calf muscles is often seen when arterial occlusion is unilateral.

Skin nutrition is also affected and hair may disappear from the lower calf and foot. The pulp of the toes may lose its normal ridging and become smooth and glossy, and the nails may become cracked and brittle.

Pressure over bony prominences can cause necrosis of skin and ulceration is not infrequent on the sides of the foot or on the heel. Where there is peripheral neuritis and anaesthesia, penetrating or trophic ulceration can occur.

Diabetic atherosclerosis

Patients with diabetes mellitus develop atherosclerosis at an earlier age than non-diabetic patients and a higher proportion of women are affected. The arterial lesions may affect the aorta, iliac or femoral arteries and cause claudication but, in most patients, the disease affects the lower popliteal and tibial arteries. The collateral circulation is poor in these distal occlusions and diabetic patients have a high incidence of ulceration and gangrene.

Diabetics are prone to develop eye and kidney complications due to disease of the smaller arteries and a similar arteritis affects the small arteries of the foot. The tissues have a poor resistance to infection which spreads rapidly in ischaemic tissues and peripheral neuritis, which is also common, may lead to trophic ulceration.

The combination of main vessel occlusion, small vessel arteritis, peripheral neuritis and infection results in a high incidence of gangrene in diabetic patients. Indeed, the spread of infection may be uncontrollable except by urgent amputation. However, the arterial lesion is usually a distal one and it is possible to perform amputation below the knee in most cases.

Thrombo-angiitis Obliterans

This condition, which is also known as Buerger's disease, is almost exclusively a disease of young males who smoke cigarettes. Although smoking is an important aetiological factor in atherosclerosis, the relationship between thrombo-angiitis obliterans and cigarette smoking is a very close one and it has been suggested that the disease is a specific consequence of smoking in young men who have a nicotine sensitivity.

This disease is relatively rare and most patients who develop occlusive vascular disease before the age of 40 have atherosclerosis rather than thrombo-angiitis. Unlike atherosclerosis, thrombo-angiitis obliterans affects the smaller arteries and progresses in such a way that the legs, and to a lesser degree the arms, appear to 'shrivel' from the digits upwards.

The clinical picture is that of peripheral ischaemia with gangrene which progresses in episodic fashion and is frequently associated with a migrating phlebitis of the superficial veins. Its ravages may be temporarily slowed or halted by sympathectomy but it tends to progress relentlessly with amputation firstly of toe or finger, then repeated amputation at higher and higher levels. Eventually the patient may have bilateral mid-thigh amputation and digital gangrene (Fig. 52).

If the patient can stop smoking, the disease may become arrested but most of these patients are compulsive smokers and are unable to stop. Sympathectomy is of value in limiting the level of amputation but the eventual prognosis is poor.

Cystic Adventitial Disease of the Popliteal Artery

This is a condition of unknown aetiology, which mainly affects males and may occur at all ages. The production of mucinous material in the wall of the popliteal artery results in compression of the lumen at the level of the knee joint and intermittent claudication is experienced when stenosis has become severe.

The diagnosis can sometimes be made from the arteriogram which shows a smooth stenosis in the popliteal artery at the level of the knee joint. At operation, the mucinous material is evacuated and the artery is repaired in whatever way the surgeon considers is best in the individual case.

CHAPTER 14
The Aortic Arch

Lesions of the aortic arch and the great vessels arising from it are relatively uncommon. Many are symptomless and others do not cause symptoms severe enough to warrant operation, so that opportunities for studying these lesions in detail are seldom obtained.

Coarctation of aorta

This is a relatively rare congenital condition in which complete canalisation of the aorta has failed to take place during development and a part of the arch or thoracic aorta has a severe constriction (Fig. 53). The blood passes through an extensive collateral

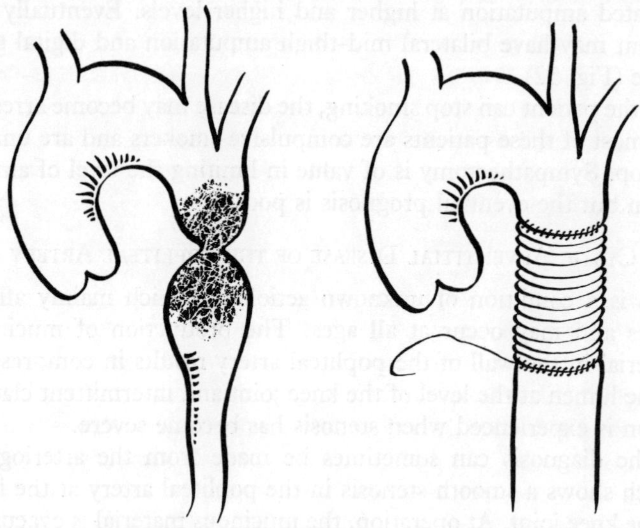

FIG. 53. Coarctation of the aorta. The narrow segment has been excised and replaced by a tubular graft.

circulation (intercostals, internal mammary) to reach the distal part of the aorta below the constriction. Hypertension occurs in the proximal aorta and its tributaries (including the cerebral vessels) as the heart attempts to force the blood through an increased peripheral resistance, and there is hypotension in the abdominal aorta and leg vessels.

Patients present with headaches or with signs of left ventricular failure. Examination reveals absence or diminution of the femoral pulses and the diagnosis is confirmed by demonstrating the constriction at aortography.

Treatment consists of excision of the constricted segment and its replacement by a tubular Dacron graft. If the arch of the aorta is affected, heart-lung bypass may be required.

Aneurysm

In the earlier part of this century, aneurysm of the aortic arch due to syphilitic aortitis was relatively common. Syphilis can now be treated adequately and few patients develop tertiary syphilis, the stage at which aortic lesions develop. Syphilitic aneurysms have therefore become quite rare. Nowadays, aneurysms of the aortic arch or thoracic aorta are uncommon and usually due to atherosclerosis. Symptoms may result from pressure on the trachea or oesophagus, erosion of the sternum, or pressure on the left recurrent laryngeal nerve which causes paralysis of the left vocal cord and consequent hoarseness. The diagnosis can usually be confirmed by an X-ray of chest which shows a large globular shadow in the mediastinum.

Treatment involves excision of the aneurysm and graft replacement with anastomosis of side channels of the graft to the great vessels if they are involved in the aneurysm. The operation can be very difficult and heart-lung bypass may be necessary.

Occlusion of the great vessels

The three main vessels arising from the aortic arch are the innominate artery which divides after a short course into the right subclavian and right common carotid arteries, the left common carotid artery and the left subclavian artery (Fig. 54).

These arteries may be affected by arterial disease of the aortic arch itself or by disease involving the first few centimetres beyond their origins from the arch. The lesion produced is either stenosis or occlusion. As the artery becomes narrower, a collateral circulation builds up through branches which anastomose with branches of the remaining patent arteries, and this collateral circulation is so extensive that occlusion can occur without symptoms.

The first indication of an occlusion may be absent pulsation in either arm noticed during routine examination—the condition called *pulseless disease*. There may be no symptoms other than a feeling of tiredness in the arm. The cerebral circulation is rarely reduced so severely as to cause symptoms.

The condition causing the occlusion may be atherosclerosis but sometimes it is due to a non-specific arteritis which can affect patients in their twenties or thirties. The cause is unknown and it is sometimes called *Takayasu's disease*, after the author who first described it.

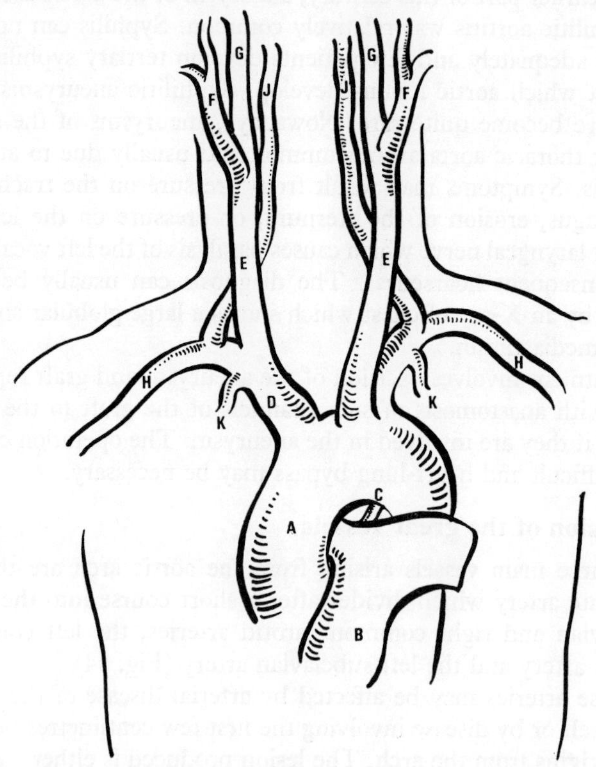

FIG. 54. The arch of the aorta and its branches. A aorta, B pulmonary artery, C ligamentum arteriosum, D innominate artery, E common carotid artery, F external carotid artery, G internal carotid artery, H subclavian artery, J vertebral artery, K internal mammary artery.

Treatment of these lesions is rarely necessary and opportunities are seldom available for studying the microscopic appearances of the arteries. Consequently, our knowledge of these conditions is incomplete.

CHAPTER 15

Arterial Occlusion in the Upper Limb

The circulation to the upper limb may be affected by any arterial lesion involving the arteries between the aortic arch and the digital arteries. In general, ischaemia is less common in the arm than in the leg but there is a larger variety of conditions causing symptoms.

Arterial occlusion or narrowing may be symptomless owing to the extensive collateral circulation available in the arm or to the double arterial pathway provided in the forearm. Ischaemia is most severe when the axillary or brachial artery is occluded because the collateral circulation at this level is less than that available in subclavian and forearm lesions. The radial and ulnar arteries take origin from the brachial artery at its bifurcation and join freely in the palm by means of the palmar arches. Blockage of one artery leads to all the blood flowing down the other and the blood supply of the hand remains normal.

Should symptoms develop, these are exercise pain (intermittent claudication), incipient or established gangrene. Claudication is felt as a tiredness in the arm when performing repetitive movements at work, or, for example, in brushing the hair. Pre-gangrenous changes are more common than actual gangrene and the changes seen in the fingers are flattening of the pulp, loss of the normal pulp ridging, painful hacks or ulceration. When ischaemia is severe, cyanosis and rest pain occur and further deterioration leads to gangrene. Gangrene is usually the 'dry' type, is rarely extensive, and is due either to multiple occlusions in the digital arteries or to sudden occlusion of a major artery caused by embolism.

Atherosclerosis

This disease may cause arterial occlusion in the arm but symptoms are rare and the condition is usually discovered during routine examination of a patient when the radial pulse is found to be weak or absent.

It may affect the major vessels arising from the aortic arch and lead to their gradual occlusion but symptoms are seldom severe owing to the extensive collateral circulation which develops. In some patients, atherosclerosis produces multiple occlusions in the digital arteries which result in the development of Raynaud's phenomenon or gangrene.

Arterial injuries

Trauma is an important cause of arterial occlusion in the upper limb and the arterial injury may be '*closed*' where the skin is unbroken or '*penetrating*' where some penetrating instrument or missile causes the injury.

The subclavian artery may occasionally be torn in severe comminuted fractures of the clavicle, the axillary artery may be stretched and torn in shoulder dislocations, and the brachial artery may be damaged in widely separated fractures of the humerus or in severe fractures and dislocations around the elbow joint. One unusual result of acute arterial damage is *Volkmann's ischaemic contracture*, which may follow injury to the brachial artery in the region of the elbow joint. In this condition, gangrene does not develop but the flexor muscles of the forearm become ischaemic and undergo replacement by fibrous tissue which contracts and produces a claw-like deformity of the hand.

Another unusual condition is thrombosis of the axillary artery caused by persistent pressure from a crutch used for many years (e.g., 20 to 30 years). This occurs in patients who have walked with the aid of a crutch instead of an artificial leg.

The treatment of arterial injury requires preliminary reduction of fractures and dislocations, with operative plating of fractures where necessary in order to stabilise the bone. The arterial injury is then explored as a matter of urgency with a view to replacement of the artery by a saphenous vein graft. If arterial continuity cannot be restored, sympathectomy may be required.

Cervical rib: subclavian thrombosis and subclavian aneurysm

A 'cervical' rib is an extra rib which articulates with the seventh cervical vertebrae behind. It may extend forwards to join the front of the first rib, but sometimes it may be only partly developed or represented by a fibrous band. The brachial plexus, subclavian artery and subclavian vein have to pass over the top of the cervical rib to reach the upper arm and symptoms of nerve, artery or vein compression may result.

The subclavian artery is compressed between the scalenus anterior muscle and the cervical rib and stenosis of the artery develops. In the course of time, one of two events may occur.

1. Thrombosis of the subclavian artery produces ischaemia without gangrene because a good collateral circulation has already developed during the stage of stenosis. Claudication may be experienced in the forearm muscles but, occasionally, thrombosis extends to involve the vertebral and carotid arteries and causes symptoms of diminished blood flow to the brain.

2. As stenosis progresses, the artery beyond the narrowed segment becomes dilated—*post-stenotic dilatation.* Continued dilatation causes an actual aneurysm which may accumulate thrombus in its sac and this may be thrown off as repeated showers of small emboli or as one large embolus. Embolisation of the smaller digital arteries may occur and give rise to Raynaud's phenomenon (see below). At any time there may be a major embolic incident with a threat of gangrene to the whole hand.

Clinically, subclavian thrombosis may present as a cold, easily tired arm, as claudication of the forearm muscles, or as an incidental finding of an absent radial pulse. A subclavian aneurysm may present as a pulsating mass lying above the clavicle, as a case of Raynaud's phenomenon, or as acute ischaemia with incipient or actual gangrene due to embolism.

The treatment varies according to the nature and severity of the circulatory deficiency. Many patients will require no treatment. In others, the neck is explored with a view to excision of the cervical rib and upper dorsal sympathectomy (p. 159) or to replace the aneurysm with a vein or Dacron graft. If embolism should occur, urgent exploration is required with a view to embolectomy.

Raynaud's phenomenon

In 1826, Raynaud described colour changes in the hand occurring in response to cold and attributed these changes to intermittent spasm of the digital arteries. Since that time, there has been argument as to whether there is a specific disease—Raynaud's disease —or merely a sequence of colour changes caused by exposure to cold and occurring as a symptom of a number of conditions—

Raynaud's phenomenon. This argument has not yet been resolved.

The characteristic colour change is a pure white colour of some or all fingers occurring on exposure to cold. This may be followed by cyanosis of the fingers before the colour returns to normal or the blanching may be followed by a fiery red stage before normal colour is restored. Some patients never show blanching but merely develop cyanotic changes on exposure to cold.

Ischaemic changes are seldom severe and usually consist of loss of the normal pulp ridging but patients with severe ischaemia may develop painful hacks, ulceration, or finger-tip gangrene.

During the stage of blanching, there is a complete shut down of the circulation through the fingers caused by severe arterial constriction. Cyanosis indicates a less severe circulatory deficiency and is due to sluggish circulation through the fingers. The tissues take up most of the oxygen carried in the slowly flowing blood, producing the deoxygenated form of haemoglobin which is blue in colour.

Raynaud's phenomenon often affects young people who have a family history of the condition but it may also occur in early or late middle age when women are more often affected than men. There are several possible underlying causes such as injury, rheumatoid arthritis or other collagen disorders, scleroderma, atherosclerosis, multiple emboli from subclavian aneurysm. In any individual case it is very difficult to determine the underlying cause and many cases appear to have no specific aetiology.

Arteriography frequently reveals extensive occlusions in the digital arteries, the palmar arteries, or the distal portions of the radial and ulnar arteries (Fig. 55). Blood has to flow through an extensive collateral circulation and the extra resistance produced by vasoconstriction in cold conditions leads to a temporary reduction or shut-down of the digital circulation.

Most patients do not deteriorate and require only reassurance. In severe cases, sympathectomy will improve the circulation but this improvement may wear off as sympathetic vasoconstrictor control is re-established through alternative pathways.

Thrombo-angiitis obliterans

Thrombo-angiitis obliterans (or Buerger's disease) in the arm is incidental to more extensive disease in the leg (Fig. 52). The distal arteries, especially of the fingers, gradually become obliterated and digital gangrene appears when the collateral circulation is inadequate to maintain viability. The first essential is to stop the patient from smoking. Sympathectomy may improve blood flow sufficiently as to limit the spread of gangrene but, very frequently, the disease results in amputation of fingers in a patient who has already lost one or both legs.

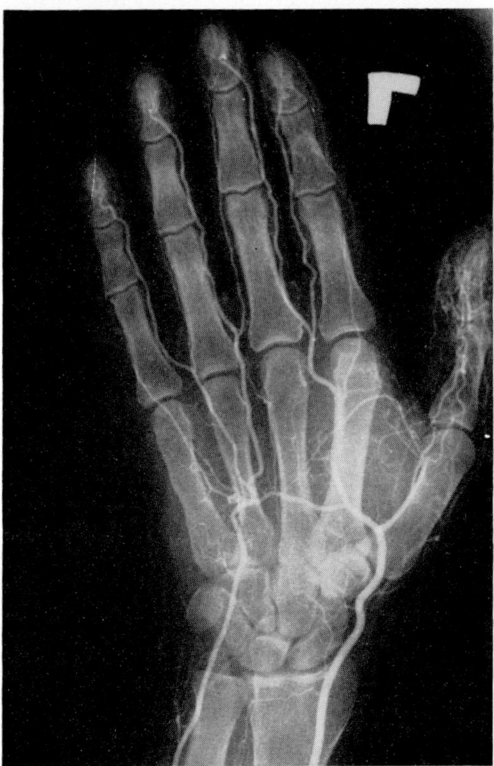

FIG. 55. Brachial arteriogram. The arterial supply to the lateral side of the index finger, the medial side of the ring and little fingers is interrupted by occlusion of the digital arteries.

To face page 124

CHAPTER 16

Lesions of the Carotid and Vertebral Arteries

The blood supply to the brain comes from the two internal carotid and the two vertebral arteries (Fig. 54) which end at the circle of Willis—a 'circle' of anastomosing arterial channels situated at the base of the brain. The internal carotid artery arises at the bifurcation of the common carotid artery in the neck and the origin of the common carotid arteries differs on the two sides, the right arising from the innominate artery and the left arising directly from the aortic arch. The vertebral arteries arise from the subclavian arteries near their origins and pass upwards in the vertebral column to reach the base of the brain posteriorly.

Cerebral ischaemia due to lesions of these arteries is unlikely to occur when only one artery is diseased and a combination of lesions is more often the cause of symptoms. These arteries may become stenosed at their origin due to atherosclerosis and progression of this disease is likely to lead to arterial occlusion in the course of time. In certain circumstances, occlusion of the internal carotid artery may produce a 'stroke' with hemiplegia. Before this serious condition has developed there may be warning symptoms indicating transient cerebral ischaemia and the diagnosis must be made at this stage for surgery to be worthwhile. When internal carotid thrombosis has occurred, no operation can restore patency to the artery as thrombosis will have extended to the inaccessible portion of artery which lies at the base of the brain in the cavernous sinus. Unilateral internal carotid occlusion, however, does not necessarily cause symptoms if the blood supply through the other three arteries is adequate.

SYMPTOMS AND SIGNS

Transient symptoms of cerebral ischaemia may occur as headache and giddiness, temporary disturbance of vision or speech, temporary facial or limb weakness. These are not diagnostic of arterial insufficiency but, when they are due to this cause, attacks are liable to occur at intervals until thrombosis produces an actual stroke.

Some patients experience 'drop attacks' in which they become unconscious and fall. These are often precipitated by rotation of the neck which causes temporary restriction of blood supply through the vertebral arteries, especially in patients with arthritic changes in the cervical spine. Examination of a patient may reveal evidence of facial or limb weakness or abnormal reflexes.

Palpation of the neck will show whether the carotid arteries are pulsating normally. Sometimes a thrill can be felt or, more commonly, auscultation will reveal a loud bruit at the carotid bifurcation in patients with carotid stenosis.

INVESTIGATION

If there is reason to suspect a vascular abnormality, an arch aortogram should be undertaken. The patient is anaesthetised, a Seldinger catheter is passed upwards from the femoral artery to the arch of the aorta, and 50 ml. of dye are forcibly injected. This will visualise the arch of the aorta and the main branches, including the four cerebral arteries. If the carotid arteries are poorly outlined, a further injection of dye given directly into the common carotid artery may help to show up the lesion. Some radiologists prefer to undertake carotid arteriography alone and only perform an arch aortogram where it is specifically indicated.

One interesting lesion which is sometimes revealed is a 'subclavian steal' (Fig. 56). When the innominate artery or either subclavian artery is occluded before the vertebral artery is given off, there is no direct blood supply to the arm. A collateral circulation may then develop from the normal side via the subclavian and vertebral arteries and the blood passes upwards, short-circuits the brain in the circle of Willis and travels down the vertebral or carotid artery of the affected side so as to reach the subclavian artery and thence the arm. This tends to reduce cerebral blood flow because the subclavian is 'stealing' blood from the brain to supply the arm. If symptoms of cerebral ischaemia occur, the condition is called the 'subclavian steal syndrome'.

TREATMENT

Symptoms may be due to reduction in blood supply or to small emboli thrown off from the diseased artery. Treatment consists of

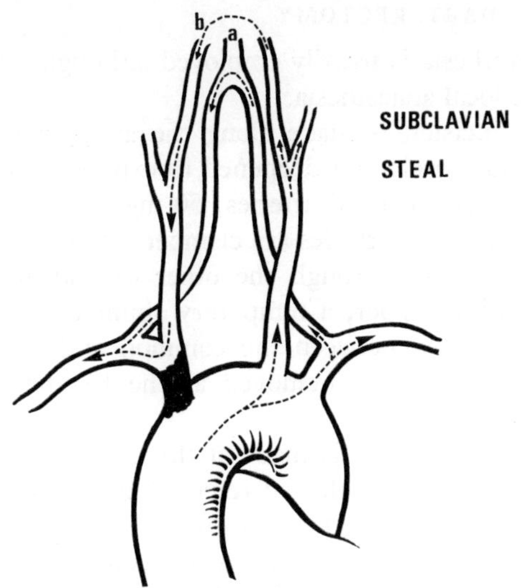

FIG. 56. Subclavian steal. The innominate artery is occluded and blood is supplied to the right arm via the vertebral arteries which unite to form the basilar artery (A) and the internal carotid arteries through the circle of Willis (B).

endarterectomy of the carotid or vertebral artery with or without insertion of a Dacron patch during closure. A technically satisfactory operation will eliminate the source of emboli and improve blood flow to the brain.

The principal difficulty in treatment is to decide when operation is justified. Operation is not possible when thrombosis has occurred so that operation must be performed at the stage of stenosis if it is to be of any value. Carotid or vertebral stenosis may be found during routine examination for other conditions caused by atherosclerosis, e.g. coronary artery thrombosis or intermittent claudication. The decision to operate or not depends to a large extent on the attitude of the surgeon who may wish to await developments or to operate in the belief that he will prevent cerebral complications.

There is no doubt that the best technical results are obtained when the lesion is operated on at an early stage but such a policy will result in some unnecessary operations being performed.

CAROTID ENDARTERECTOMY

General anaesthesia is usually employed although some surgeons prefer to use local anaesthesia.

A vertical incision is made along the anterior border of the sterno-mastoid muscle and deepened to expose the common, external, and internal carotid arteries; 50 mg. of heparin are given intravenously and the arteries are clamped. If there is any indication that blood flow through the other carotid artery and the vertebral arteries is poor, a temporary shunt can be inserted to maintain blood flow between the common and internal carotid arteries, the shunt being removed as the last few stitches are inserted.

A longitudinal incision is made at the carotid bifurcation, the thickened intima is split off and removed from the common and internal arteries and care is taken to ensure that there is no residual intimal flap in the internal carotid which could be stripped up by the flow of blood. The lesion in the internal carotid is usually confined to the first centimetre and the artery beyond is of normal calibre.

The incision is closed with a continuous suture of 4/O or 5/O silk or other non-absorbable material. If it seems likely that this suture would narrow the artery, a patch of Dacron is inserted to prevent narrowing. The clamps are then removed, the heparin is reversed (p. 143) and the wound is sutured.

Post-operative recovery is rapid and complications are rare.

CHAPTER 17

Disease of the Visceral Arteries: Intestinal Ischaemia

The alimentary tract is supplied by three main arteries—the coeliac axis, the superior mesenteric and the inferior mesenteric arteries (Fig. 57), which supply the upper, middle and lower parts of the alimentary tract respectively. Narrowing or blockage of these arteries will give rise to ischaemia of bowel which may be acute or chronic depending on the rapidity with which events take place.

The syndromes produced vary between the sudden catastrophic gangrene of large parts of the alimentary tract and more subtle disorders of absorption and digestion. Recognition of the latter is very recent and elucidation of the various arterial lesions and their symptom patterns requires further investigation at the present time.

The Superior Mesenteric Artery

Acute intestinal ischaemia

Sudden occlusion of the superior mesenteric artery cuts off the blood supply to the small intestine, the ascending colon and part of the transverse colon. If the circulation is not restored within a few hours, gangrene of bowel and peritonitis will develop and urgent removal of all dead bowel is the only means of saving the patient. There are two main causes—embolism and thrombosis.

Mesenteric embolism. The material which plugs the artery is usually thrombus derived from one of a number of sources (p. 139). The embolus may be single or multiple, or may break up into fragments after impact.

When the artery is plugged, the arterial tree beyond the block empties. Within a matter of hours, it refills with blood as nature attempts to restore circulation through other channels. Alternatively, blood comes back from the veins to fill the empty arteries. When this blood thromboses in the arteries, it is impossible to restore normal circulation and gangrene of bowel is inevitable.

Mesenteric thrombosis. The usual cause is atherosclerosis which affects the origin or the first few centimetres of the artery and causes progressive narrowing. At some stage, thrombosis occurs with complete blockage of the artery. During the stage of stenosis, anastomoses between the three visceral arteries may have enlarged sufficiently so as to maintain a reasonable blood supply to the affected bowel after thrombosis of one artery but, in most cases, this collateral circulation is inadequate and acute ischaemia of bowel results.

The sequence of events in the distal arteries is similar to that in

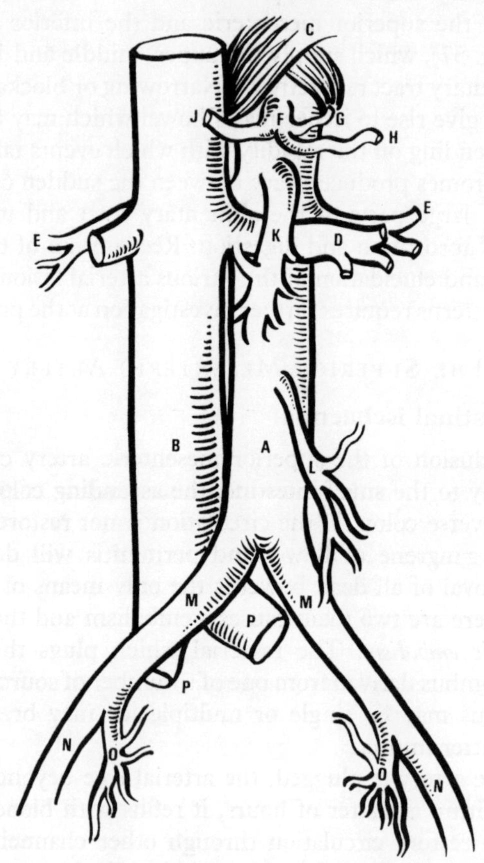

FIG. 57. The abdominal aorta and its branches. A aorta, B inferior vena cava, C crura of diaphragm, D renal vein, E renal artery, F coeliac axis, G left gastric artery, H splenic artery, J hepatic artery, K superior mesenteric artery, L inferior mesenteric artery, M common iliac artery, N external iliac artery, O internal iliac artery, P common iliac vein.

embolism and extensive arterial thrombosis leads to gangrene within several hours of onset.

CLINICAL FEATURES

The clinical features of acute infarction of bowel due to embolism or thrombosis are essentially the same.

A middle-aged or elderly patient who may have evidence of a source of emboli, or have evidence of atherosclerosis elsewhere (e.g., previous coronary thrombosis, intermittent claudication, etc.) develops abdominal pain. The onset of symptoms may be acute with severe pain and shock due to rapid blood loss and toxaemia but, in many cases, the onset is insidious and the pain is ill-defined with only gradual deterioration in the patient's general condition. Vomiting is common but diarrhoea and the passage of a blood-stained stool are not.

The patient's condition deteriorates due to loss of blood and fluid into the bowel and the abdomen is tender. Distension appears later and vomiting becomes frequent and faeculent as gangrene of bowel and peritonitis ensue.

TREATMENT

It is often difficult to make the proper diagnosis at an early stage especially when the onset is insidious. Operation is usually undertaken too late to save the patient. In most cases the whole of the small intestine and part of the transverse colon is gangrenous and excision would leave too little bowel for the patient to survive.

In some patients, gangrene of the bowel is limited in extent and resection of bowel may be possible with survival of the patient. If operation has been performed early enough, it is sometimes possible to remove the embolus or to restore blood supply to the artery by arterial grafting, but success by these methods is rare.

Chronic intestinal ischaemia

Reduction in the blood supply through one or more of the visceral arteries leads to the development of a collateral circulation through anastomoses with the other arteries which may or may not succeed in supplying sufficient blood to the bowel to allow normal digestion and absorption. If the alternative blood supply is adequate, no symptoms will result and the patient may remain healthy indefinitely. However, it is usual to find that more than one of the three main arteries is involved when atherosclerosis is the cause, and that an adequate collateral circulation does not develop. The chronic deficiency in blood supply to the bowel then leads to a pattern of symptoms which reflect the inability of the small bowel to digest and absorb food properly.

The principal symptom is pain which occurs after each meal, especially large meals. This time relationship to meals is similar to that of ulcer pain but, unlike ulcers which heal and give free spells from dyspeptic symptoms, ischaemic pain tends to occur after every meal. It has been described as 'intestinal angina' because the pain is brought on by the stress of having to digest a big meal.

The other important feature is loss of weight due to small meals and poor absorption and the patient can lose weight quite rapidly. Another symptom of poor absorption may be the passage of bulky stools caused by excessive loss of fat in the faeces.

The importance of recognising this stage of chronic ischaemia lies in the fact that many patients subsequently develop thrombosis and acute infarction of bowel, which is associated with a high fatality rate. Therefore, if the condition can be diagnosed and treated at the stage of chronic ischaemia, the patient's life may be saved.

Diagnosis of chronic ischaemia is difficult because it is an uncommon condition which is often atypical in its symptomatology. It should be suspected when a middle aged patient complains of persistent abdominal pain associated with severe weight loss. Auscultation of the epigastrium may reveal the presence of a bruit produced by a stenosed artery. Diagnosis can be confirmed by an aortogram performed in the lateral position so that the bowel arteries are seen in profile (Fig. 58). In the normal A-P view, the origins of the three main arteries are superimposed on the aortic shadow and narrowing of the first centimetre or two of the arteries cannot be seen.

TREATMENT

The only possible treatment is operation to restore blood supply to the bowel. This can be done in several ways, the method used depending on the conditions found at operation and on the preference of the surgeon. He can use a bypass vein or Dacron graft between the aorta and superior mesenteric artery, he can reimplant the patent part of the artery into the aorta, or he may perform an endarterectomy of the occluded portion.

THE COELIAC AXIS

This artery supplies the stomach, part of the duodenum, liver, spleen and pancreas. Sudden occlusion by embolism or thrombosis is rare. The commonest lesion is a narrowing of the artery caused by atherosclerosis which usually affects the superior mesenteric artery as well, and symptoms due to disease of the latter overshadow the changes produced in the coeliac axis.

In the last few years, constriction of the coeliac axis (and sometimes also the superior mesenteric) due to peri-arterial fibrosis or compression by the median arcuate ligament of the diaphragm has been described. The symptoms produced are largely those of abdominal discomfort and loss of weight, and an epigastric bruit is usually present. The finding of the bruit is not necessarily diagnostic, as abdominal bruits can be heard in coeliac axis or superior mesenteric stenosis, renal artery stenosis, aortic bifurcation stenosis, and aortic aneurysm.

The diagnosis is confirmed by lateral aortography (Fig. 58). If the patient's symptoms are severe enough to warrant operation, the coeliac axis is explored with a view to division of the median arcuate ligament or removal of the constricting fibrous tissue. At the present time, the full clinical significance of this condition has not been elucidated.

THE INFERIOR MESENTERIC ARTERY

This artery supplies the left half of the colon and upper rectum. Occlusion or stenosis seldom give rise to symptoms because the left side of the colon has a large marginal artery running along its mesenteric border and an adequate blood supply from the superior mesenteric artery is guaranteed so long as this anastomotic artery is intact.

Occasionally, acute blockage due to embolism or thrombosis may give rise to gangrene of the left side of the colon and the serious nature of this condition is similar to that of acute infarction of the small intestine. In other patients, occlusion of the inferior mesenteric artery produces chronic ischaemia of a segment of colon which develops chronic inflammatory changes or stricture. This condition is called *ischaemic colitis.*

CHAPTER 18

Renal Artery Stenosis and Hypertension

Following Goldblatt's demonstration in 1934 that ischaemia of the kidney produced by constricting the renal artery could cause hypertension, attempts were made to explain hypertension in terms of renal disease. No constant association between hypertension and renal disease could be demonstrated but occasional dramatic cures followed the removal of a unilateral diseased kidney. With the advent of aortography, it became possible to study the renal arteries and it was soon found that a number of patients with hypertension had stenosis of one or both renal arteries. These cases, however, were disappointingly few and corrective surgery proved variable in its results.

It is now acknowledged that renal artery stenosis causing hypertension is relatively uncommon and accounts for only 3 to 5 per cent of the hypertensive population. It can occur at all ages and is caused by a number of unrelated conditions.

The commonest cause is probably atherosclerosis and many of these patients are in their forties. A rather unusual cause of arterial disease, fibro-muscular dysplasia, is responsible for most of the remaining cases and this affects a younger age group. Other causes are rare, e.g., congenital, Takayasu's arteritis.

Investigation

When a patient is found to have hypertension, i.e., persistent elevation of both systolic and diastolic pressure to above 160/100 mm. mercury at rest, the decision must be made as to whether or not to undertake investigation. In most cases, the age of the patient or his general fitness will preclude investigation and treatment with antihypertensive drugs will be preferable. If the patient is fit a number of investigations can be undertaken to demonstrate the presence of renal artery stenosis but not all need be done in each patient. These investigations are intravenous pyelogram, isotope renogram, split renal function studies, and aortography.

The initial screening test carried out in all patients is a dehydration *intravenous pyelogram* with films taken in rapid sequence. When unilateral renal artery stenosis is present, dye excretion on the pyelogram is delayed on the affected side due to reduced glomerular filtration and, as there is also increased reabsorption of water in the renal tubules, the concentration of dye in the renal pelvis is increased giving an appearance of 'spastic' renal calyces. On the intravenous pyelogram therefore, delayed excretion of dye giving an intense dye shadow on one side is presumptive evidence of unilateral renal artery stenosis on that side.

Other lesions may be revealed by the pyelogram. There may be an absence of dye excretion on one side due to a non-functioning kidney affected by severe chronic pyelonephritis, pyonephrosis or other lesion. If the other kidney is healthy as shown by renal function studies and retrograde pyelography, nephrectomy may be indicated and may lead to relief of hypertension. In some cases, the pyelogram will show bilateral renal disease, when it is unlikely that surgery will be helpful.

If equipment is available, the next screening test is the *isotope renogram*. A measured amount of radioactive isotope (2 to 8 microcuries of radiohippuran) is injected intravenously following 20 hours dehydration and the rate of uptake and excretion by the kidney is measured by Geiger counters placed over each kidney (Fig. 59). The counting rate obtained due to uptake and excretion of the isotope by the kidney gives a measure of kidney function and

TABLE II

Howard test (divided renal function studies)

Note the low volume, low sodium and high urea and creatinine concentrations in the urine collected from the left kidney, when left renal artery stenosis was present.

	Right kidney	Left kidney
Urine volume (ml.)	38·0	9·5
Sodium	102·0	87·0
Urea	0·48	1·04
Creatinine	12·8	47·5

alterations in the shape of the curve are of value in the diagnosis of renal artery stenosis (Fig. 60).

Positive evidence from these two tests is sufficient to justify proceeding with aortography. Some investigators prefer to undertake *split function studies* (the Howard test) before aortography while others utilise this test only in patients where there is some doubt as to diagnosis or the degree of abnormal function present.

In this test, the patient is given an intravenous infusion of ureaphil to force a diuresis and the urine is collected from each kidney over a fixed period and then analysed. There is a reduction in urine volume, a reduction in sodium and chloride concentration, and an increase in creatinine and urea concentration from a kidney affected by renal artery stenosis as compared with the normal side (Table II).

Aortography is required in order to reveal the outlines of the renal arteries (Fig. 61). A stenosed artery usually shows a constriction near its origin with post-stenotic dilatation beyond, but sometimes the arterial lesion is seen to extend into the branches. During the nephrogram phase of the aortogram, the dye passes through the parenchyma of the kidney and gives a shadow which permits measurement of kidney size. When atherosclerosis is present, irregularity or tortuosity of the aorta and iliac arteries can be seen.

If the arterial lesion affects most of the renal artery or its branches, surgery is not possible. If the kidney is small, it may be best to undertake nephrectomy. If the kidney appears to be of reasonable size and the arterial lesion is unilateral and localised, exploration is indicated with a view to conservative surgery whose aim is to restore normal blood flow to the kidney.

Pre-operative management

The patient's fitness is assessed by routine clinical examination supplemented by haemoglobin estimation, X-ray of chest, electrocardiogram, urea and electrolytes and creatinine clearance test. Four to six pints of blood are cross-matched and antibiotic cover (p. 148) is commenced. A naso-gastric tube is passed in the ward and a special note is taken of the pre-operative blood pressure. An indwelling catheter is inserted into the bladder prior to operation to facilitate accurate measurement of urine output during and after operation.

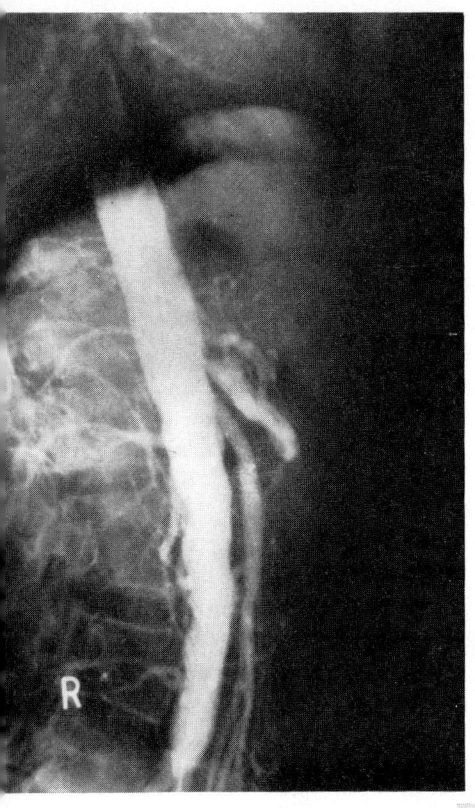

FIG. 58. Lateral aortogram of the abdominal aorta. The coeliac axis is narrowed at its origin whereas the superior mesenteric artery below it is of reasonable calibre.

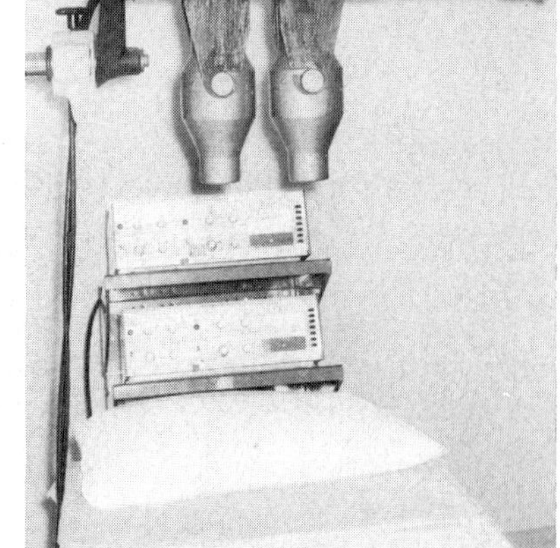

IG. 59. Isotope renography. The two eiger counters are lowered and placed ne over each kidney, and the rate of isope excretion is measured on the scintiltion counters at the head of the couch.

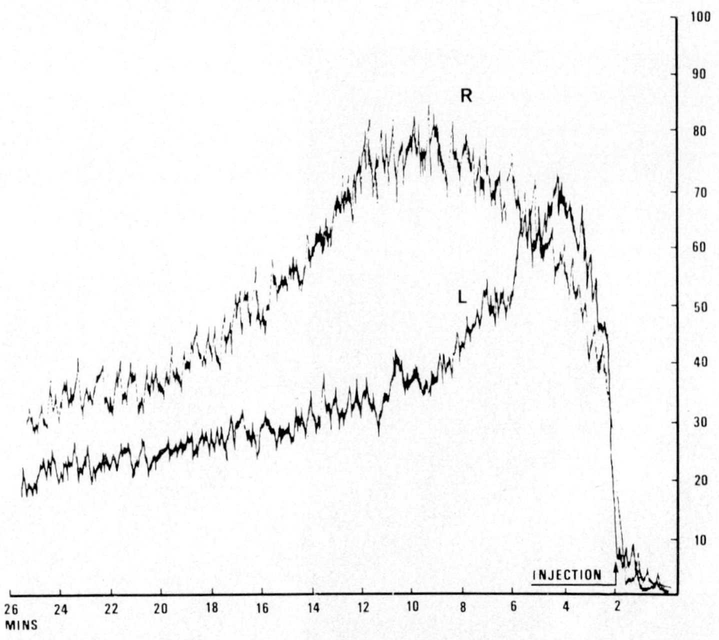

FIG. 60. Isotope renogram tracing. This is read from right to left. The curve obtained from the left kidney (L) is normal with a rapidly attained peak at 3 min. followed by a rapid fall. The right kidney (R) shows a slower uptake with a delayed peak at 8 min. and a slower fall.

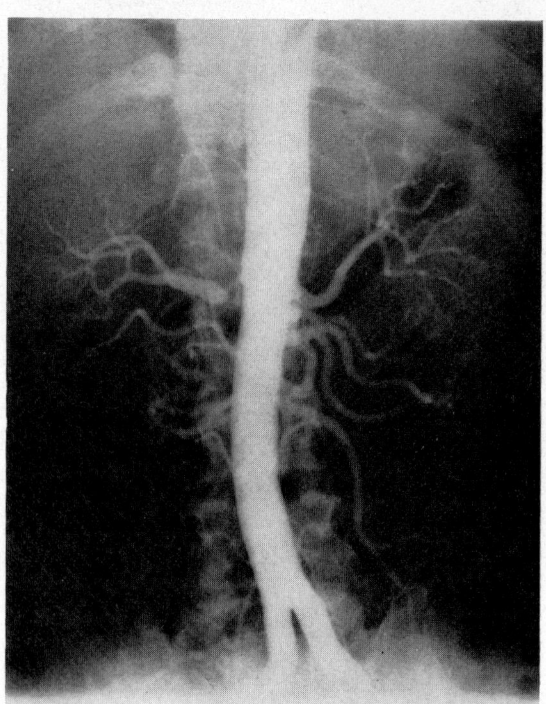

FIG. 61. Stenosis of the right renal artery. There is severe narrowing of the commencement of the artery and post-stenotic dilatation distally.

Operation

The best incision is a transverse incision, convex upwards, situated well above the umbilicus and curving downwards into the flank. The hepatic or splenic flexure of the colon is mobilised and turned downwards and dissection gives access to the aorta between the level of the renal veins and the aortic bifurcation. The renal artery is found lying behind the vein and, on the right side, the inferior vena cava has to be mobilised by division of its tributaries in order to expose the proximal portion of the renal artery. The amount of dissection required depends on the method of revascularisation adopted. If the condition is atherosclerotic and thrombo-endarterectomy is to be employed, the aorta must be dissected above the renal arteries to allow it to be clamped. If a bypass graft is to be inserted, only the aorta below the left renal vein need be dissected free and clamped. When dissection is complete, 50 mg. heparin are injected intravenously.

Revascularisation is performed either (1) by incising the artery to remove the thickened intima and closing the incision with a vein or Dacron patch, (2) by dividing the artery at the site of the post-stenotic dilatation and reimplanting the artery into the aorta or (3) by attaching a saphenous vein or single Dacron graft to the aorta and renal artery as a bypass. This bypass graft may be attached to the side of the renal artery or the artery can be divided and an end-to-end anastomosis performed.

When the anastomoses are sound, the clamps are released to allow blood to flow into the kidney and the heparin is reversed (p. 143). As the kidney should not be cut off from its arterial flow for more than one hour, there is a limit to the operative time available but this margin is more than adequate. When haemostasis is satisfactory, the wound is closed with a vacuum drain to the site of operation.

Post-operative management

Post-operative care is the same as for aorto-iliac operations (p. 150). Mannitol or frusemide (Lasix) is given as required to stimulate urine secretion, blood pressure is recorded hourly for 24 hours then intermittently as indicated, and gastric suction and intravenous fluids are continued until the paralytic ileus resolves (p. 152). The catheter is removed on the second day and the patient is out of bed on the third or fourth day when the ileus has settled. He can usually be dismissed home after 12 or 14 days.

Complications

These are relatively few and are similar to those following aorto-iliac operations (p. 151).

Occasionally, the graft will thrombose at an early stage. The patient then requires further operation to remove the graft and the useless kidney—'secondary nephrectomy'.

Results

When the kidneys have not been severely damaged by the hypertension, the blood pressure will revert to normal in about two-thirds of cases if the restoration of blood flow has been technically satisfactory. Patients whose blood pressure does not return to normal may show a reduction in pressure and the residual hypertension can often be controlled by antihypertensive drugs.

CHAPTER 19

Embolism of the Peripheral Arteries

Embolism is the obstruction or occlusion of a vessel by detached thrombus or other foreign material. The vessel is usually an artery as the flow of blood is in the direction of diminishing size but it may also occur in lymph vessels (e.g. tumour emboli).

Types of embolism

Systemic embolism. The usual obstructing material is a thrombus derived from one of a number of sources which passes out in the systemic arterial circulation to lodge in the arteries of the brain, limbs, or abdominal viscera.

Pulmonary embolism. In this condition, thrombus is derived from the veins of the leg or pelvis and passes through the right side of the heart to lodge in the pulmonary arteries. Sudden death or pulmonary infarct may result.

Paradoxical embolism. In this rare type, thrombus derived from the systemic veins passes to the right atrium, then enters the left atrium through a patent foramen ovale (p. 50) and is pumped out by the left ventricle into the systemic circulation.

Other materials may act as emboli, e.g. air embolism, fat embolism, lymphatic embolism.

Common sources of emboli

Systemic emboli may arise in a variety of situations. (1) The atrium is a possible site in auricular fibrillation. When contraction of the atrium is incoordinated and inadequate, thrombus may form in the atrial appendage or on the wall of the atrium and may be dislodged by a forcible beat of the atrium or during a heart operation. An embolic incident may sometimes be precipitated when the patient is given quinidine to convert his fibrillation or digoxin to control it. (2) In coronary artery thrombosis, thrombus may form on the endocardium at the site of an infarct, and pieces of this thrombus may separate as emboli. (3) When an atherosclerotic plaque calcifies and ulcerates, thrombus may form on the surface of the plaque and later become detached as an embolus. (4) In subacute bacterial endocarditis, bacteria can lodge in valves distorted by rheumatic disease and thrombus appears on the fringe of the valve as 'vegetations'. Valve movement may dislodge these vegetations and these emboli are potentially able to cause infection at the site of lodgment—mycotic (infected) emboli. (5) The thrombus which forms on the wall of an aneurysm (e.g., abdominal or subclavian aneurysm) may become detached. (6) Thrombus formation can occur on artificial heart valves and lead to emboli—hence the need for anticoagulants after operation. (7) Paradoxical emboli. (p. 139).

Effects of embolism

When an embolus enters the systemic arterial circulation, it may lodge in any of the peripheral arteries. The site of lodgment depends to some extent on the size of the embolus which is carried along by the flowing blood until it impacts. Sometimes it breaks up on impact and the fragments pass onwards to block the artery lower down or to block a number of smaller arteries. If this should happen, the patient's symptoms can improve as the block of a major artery is followed by the blockage of smaller less important ones.

When the embolus impacts, the blood in the artery beyond the embolus may clot (consecutive clot) or the blood in the artery distal to the plug is squeezed out and the affected tissues become pale and bloodless. In some situations, a collateral circulation through side channels has already developed and the tissues beyond the site of embolism are supplied with a reduced flow sufficient to prevent necrosis or death of tissue although symptoms of inadequate circulation may appear (e.g., intermittent claudication).

If the plugged artery is the only source of blood supply to the tissue affected, e.g., is an 'end-artery', or if no collateral circulation develops, blood will accumulate in the distal arteries by back flow from the veins or by trickling through inadequate side channels. This thromboses within 10 to 12 hours leading to widespread and irreversible blockage of the arterial circulation and death of the organ or tissue follows. In some organs, e.g., liver or spleen, an infarct is produced and this is eventually replaced by fibrous tissue. If pathogenic bacteria invade the dead tissue, gangrene will result (e.g., limbs, bowel) and operative removal of the dead tissue by amputation becomes necessary.

Symptoms and signs

These vary according to the organ affected. When embolism occurs in a leg, the patient usually experiences pain due to the acute ischaemia which results. The leg becomes pale and cold, the muscles are deprived of their blood supply and become paralysed, and anaesthesia of the toes, foot, or leg will be present.

The site of embolism can be deduced from the pulse pattern (i.e., the site is beyond the most distal pulsating artery) and from the level of coldness, paralysis and anaesthesia.

Common sites of embolism in the leg are at the aortic bifurcation where a saddle embolus blocks the orifices of the common iliac arteries and causes bilateral ischaemia, the common iliac bifurcation, the common femoral artery, the adductor canal and opening and the popliteal bifurcation. Emboli are frequently multiple and more than one of these arteries may be blocked.

If the embolus is not removed, the leg becomes livid and blue and gangrene develops. If there is doubt as to viability of the leg, the presence of anaesthesia and its extent are the best guides in determining whether the leg will survive or not.

Treatment

Removal of the embolus by operation within 10 to 12 hours usually results in complete recovery of the tissues. Embolectomy is also worthwhile even after this time interval if the collateral circulation has been sufficient to prevent gangrene.

When the diagnosis of embolism is made, the surgeon is immediately informed, 2 to 4 pints of whole blood are cross-matched, 100 mg. (10,000 International Units) of heparin are given intravenously and urgent operation is arranged. If the patient is not fit for a general anaesthetic, operation can be performed quite satisfactorily under local anaesthesia.

Operation has been greatly simplified by the use of a balloon catheter—the Fogarty catheter (Fig. 62). Embolism in a leg is dealt with as follows: the common femoral artery is exposed in the groin under general or local anaesthesia and is occluded by a clamp just below the inguinal ligament (Fig. 63). The superficial and deep femoral arteries are also occluded by clamps. An incision is made in the common femoral artery opposite the origin of the deep femoral artery and the top clamp is released briefly to confirm that there is free flow down from the aorta. If blood does not squirt out, the Fogarty catheter is passed up into the aorta, the balloon is blown up and thrombus is extracted by pulling the distended balloon downwards. When thrombus has been removed from the proximal vessel, it is reclamped and the catheter is passed down the superficial femoral artery as far as it will go. The balloon is again inflated and thrombus is extracted by withdrawing the catheter. The procedure is repeated until no more can be extracted and the deep artery is then cleared by a similar manoeuvre.

The artery is sutured with 4/0 or 5/0 non-absorbable suture material. The distal clamps are removed first to expel air through the incision and then the proximal clamp is removed. The wound is closed when haemostasis is satisfactory. The leg should rapidly

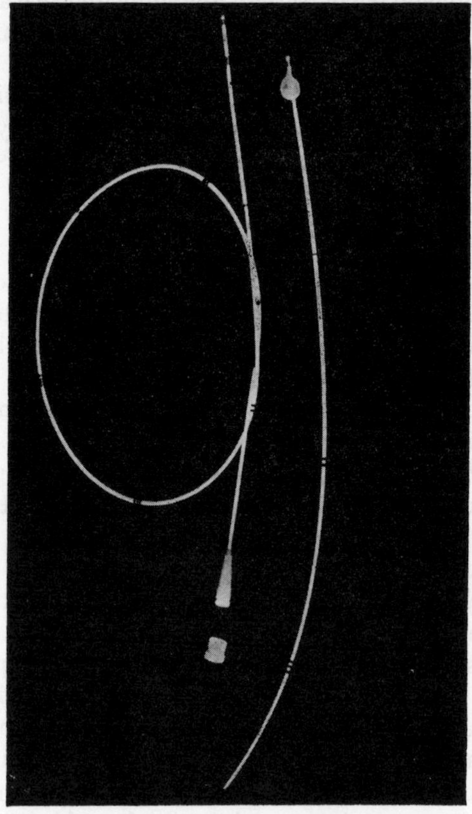

FIG. 62. Fogarty catheter—inflated and uninflated.

regain normal colour and sometimes ankle pulsation will return almost immediately. The anticoagulant effect of heparin is reversed by injecting protamine sulphate intravenously (1 mg. protamine sulphate = 1 mg. heparin) and the patient returns to the ward.

The only immediate post-operative instruction is to encourage movement of the leg. When the patient has fully recovered a day or two later, oral anticoagulants should be commenced in order to reduce the risk of recurrent emboli.

Results of operation

The time lapse between the onset of embolism and operation is crucial in determining the success of operation. When embolectomy is undertaken within 8 to 12 hours, restoration of normal blood flow is usually achieved and can be confirmed by the return of arterial pulsation in the posterior tibial and dorsalis pedis arteries. When small portions of thrombus have passed into the tibial arteries, some residual arterial blockage may remain but viability of the leg should be assured if the arterial tree has been cleared down to the popliteal bifurcation.

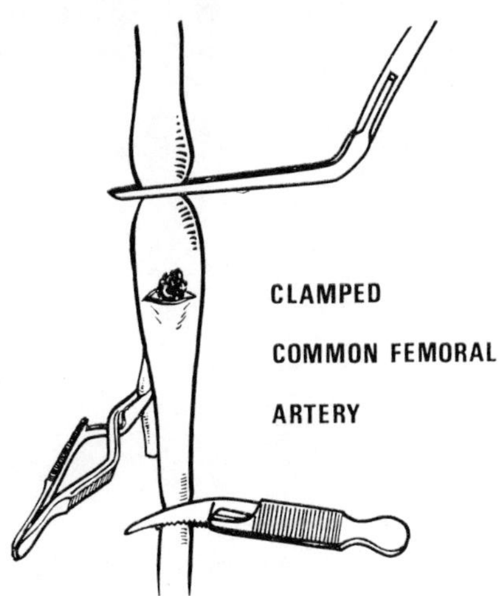

FIG. 63. Embolectomy. The common, superficial and deep femoral arteries have been clamped. A transverse incision has been made in the common femoral artery and a portion of clot has been extruded.

Late embolectomy up to 14 days after the embolic incident is possible provided that a collateral blood flow has maintained patency of the distal arteries. After two weeks, any residual thrombus in the arteries becomes organised and restoration of arterial patency can only be achieved by a formal arterial reconstruction.

When the distal arteries and veins become occluded by widespread thrombosis, embolectomy will fail and amputation will be necessary.

CHAPTER 20

Techniques in Peripheral Arterial Surgery

Although methods of arterial suture were described by Carrel in 1908 and lumbar sympathectomy was introduced in 1925, arterial operations were relatively rare until Gross, Bill and Pierce showed in 1949 that a length of diseased aorta could be replaced by a homograft, i.e., an aorta taken from a cadaver. Homografts were used until experiments with tubes of cloth and other synthetic materials led to the introduction of Teflon and Dacron in 1957 and 1958. The use of saphenous vein for bypass grafting in the femoro-popliteal segment was introduced by Kunlin in 1951, although saphenous vein replacement of a popliteal aneurysm had been successfully performed by Lexer in 1912 and Hogarth Pringle in 1913.

The two basic techniques for restoring blood flow to a leg when the main artery has become occluded due to atherosclerosis are to core out the thickened inner layer of the artery, thrombo-endarterectomy, or to bypass the occlusion by suturing a replacement artery, vein or fabric graft to the patent vessel above and below the block. The success of both methods requires that the artery and its branches below the block are patent and able to accept the increased blood flow. If this 'run-off' is inadequate blood flow will be too sluggish in the graft and thrombosis will lead to failure of the operation.

Thrombo-endarterectomy. In an atherosclerotic vessel, it is usually possible to find a place of cleavage between the thickened inner lining of the artery and the outer coat. This can be exploited at operation by separating the inner and outer coats with an arterial stripper (Fig. 64) over the length of the blocked segment. The core can then be removed leaving a patent tube whose wall is the original outer coat of the artery.

This method gives best results when the artery is large (e.g., aorta and iliac arteries), when the occluded segment is short, and when the intima is easily split from the media. Extensive calcification or inflammatory changes in the artery may make thrombo-

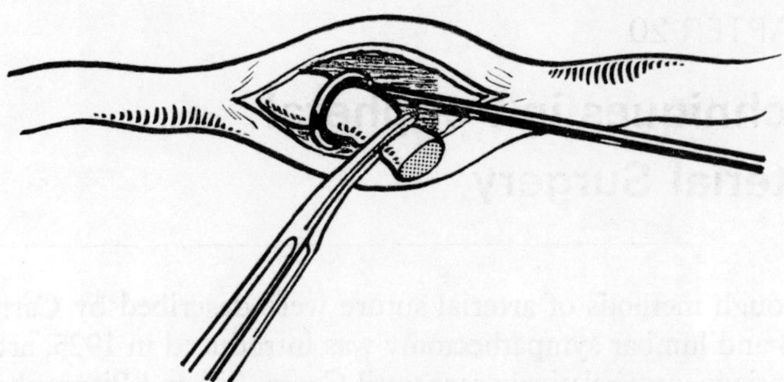

FIG. 64. Thrombo-endarterectomy. A longitudinal incision has been made in the artery. The thickened intima has been separated and divided and a ring stripper is being passed down the artery to core out the intima.

endarterectomy impossible. If satisfactory conditions are not attainable, it is preferable to undertake bypass grafting.

Incomplete removal of the intima may leave ragged tags in the rebored segment which will favour thrombosis and cause a recurrence of occlusion. Another technical difficulty is to know when to stop stripping distally because the thickened intima extends down the artery beyond the level at which operation is undertaken. Care must be taken to avoid leaving a loose flap of intima which could be stripped up by the flow of blood and cause further blockage.

Bypass grafting. As experience of arterial surgery accumulates and results are assessed, some methods of bypass grafting have been discarded because of early thrombosis or late dilatation of the graft. In patients with incipient gangrene, operative methods which give a short term result may be acceptable although normally the surgeon prefers a method which gives a reasonable long term success.

The materials available are homografts, synthetic tubes and saphenous vein. Homografts are not often used because of the difficulty of obtaining and storing suitable material and because the graft, once implanted, tends to become dilated and aneurysmal a few years later.

Synthetic fibres of Teflon or Dacron are knitted or woven into seamless straight or Y-shaped tubes (bifurcation graft) (Fig. 65). Blood clots in the interstices of the graft and is replaced by fibrous tissue which grows through and around the graft. It is thus in-

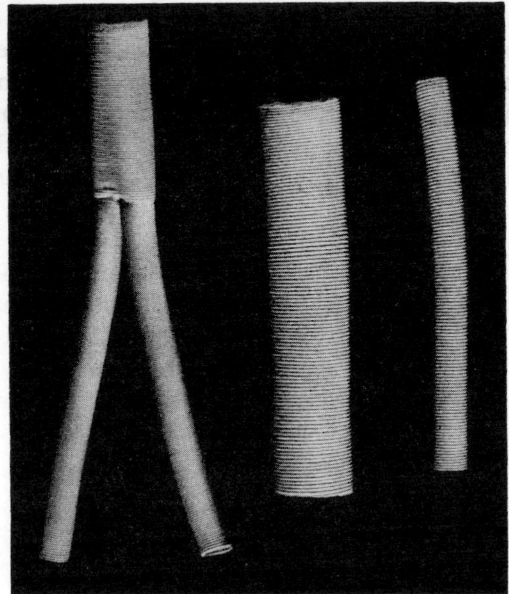

FIG. 65. Woven Dacron bifurcation and single tubular grafts

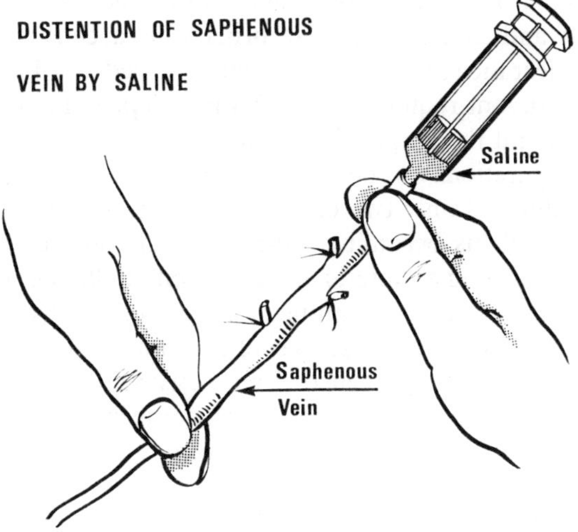

FIG. 66. Distension of the saphenous vein.

corporated into the body tissues and becomes lined by a layer of cells similar to normal endothelium. These grafts are used in aorto-iliac operations because they are readily available in different sizes and give a high success rate. They are unsuitable for femoro-popliteal operations because most of them thrombose within a year at this level and bending of the tube caused by hip or knee flexion leads to detachment of the pseudo-intimal lining and eventual thrombosis.

Saphenous vein is the material of choice in femoro-popliteal surgery and only occasionally is it found to be too small or too varicose. The vein is removed, its tributaries tied, and it is distended by forcible injection of saline to increase its diameter (Fig. 66). It is then reversed because otherwise the valves would prevent the downward flow of blood and it is sutured to patent main artery above and below the occlusion.

Aorto-iliac Operations

PRE-OPERATIVE

When the decision to operate has been made and the patient has accepted, arrangements are made for certain investigations and the patient's fitness is assessed by a physician and anaesthetist. X-ray of chest, electrocardiogram, and haemoglobin estimation are performed. Renal function is assessed by measurement of the blood urea and, if necessary, by urinary urea concentration or creatinine clearance tests. Arrangements are made for blood transfusion, the amount required (4 to 10 units) depending on the type of operation and the surgeon's technique.

These preparations can be made on an out-patient basis and the patient is admitted only two days before operation so as to minimise the risk of his becoming a carrier of the hospital staphylococcus. Prophylactic antibiotic (e.g., cloxacillin 500 mg. 6-hourly) is commenced before and continued for one week post-operatively. The patient is shaved from the level of the nipples to the knees and the umbilicus is carefully cleaned. A naso-gastric tube is introduced in the ward and an indwelling Foley catheter is introduced into the bladder after anaesthesia has been induced.

OPERATION

During operation, the anaesthetist controls the volume of blood replacement necessary by measuring the amount in the suction bottle and by assessing the loss in swabs or abdominal packs. Pulse rate and blood pressure are charted and central venous pressure may be measured by means of a catheter in the external jugular vein. Where the equipment is available, pulse rate, arterial pressure, central venous pressure and electrocardiogram may be monitored continuously on a multi-channel recorder. Urinary output is measured in a graduated cylinder connected to the in-dwelling catheter. Ringer-lactate solution is given intravenously to maintain kidney output. If urine secretion drops when the aorta is clamped, 100 ml. of 20 per cent mannitol are given rapidly into the intravenous drip.

Adequate operative exposure is necessary in order to obtain proper control of the aorta and iliac arteries and to permit operation in a dry field. This usually requires an incision from xiphisternum to symphysis pubis either in the midline or to one side of the midline (paramedian incision). Sometimes a transverse incision curving above the umbilicus is used to expose the aorta or renal arteries. The small intestine is retracted and packed off under the right wound flap or brought outside the abdomen and encased in a plastic intestinal bag. The transverse colon is packed off in the left upper abdomen.

The peritoneum to the left of the mesentery of the small bowel is incised vertically where it lies in front of the aorta, and the aorta and iliac arteries are exposed as far as necessary, care being taken to avoid damage to the large thin walled veins, the inferior vena cava and common iliac veins. When the surgeon has decided upon the type of reconstruction necessary the aorta above is occluded with a De Bakey or other clamp and the iliac and other tributaries are occluded using tapes, bulldog clamps or other methods which will not damage the vessel (Fig. 47). Thrombo-endarterectomy is performed or a bypass graft sutured in position (Fig. 67). The suture material used is non-absorbable 3/0 or 4/0 and the tendency now is to use synthetic fibres woven into a fine strand. A continuous suture is employed and, if there is a gap in the suture line which leaks when the clamps are partially released, additional interrupted sutures are inserted as necessary.

If a bypass bifurcation graft has been inserted, the distal ends of the graft may be sewn end-to-end to the common iliac arteries or end-to-side to the external iliac or common femoral arteries.

Exposure of the common femoral is made through a separate groin incision and is technically easier than suture to the external iliac artery.

When the actual operative procedure has been completed, the distal clamps are released first to expel air through the suture line then all clamps are released. Loss of blood is not severe if the surgical technique has been meticulous and if woven grafts are used. Knitted grafts tend to allow leakage at this stage if they have not been adequately pre-clotted, i.e., immersed in blood which is allowed to clot in the pores of the graft.

Many surgeons use heparin either systematically (50 mg.) or by injecting 10 mg. in saline down each leg before application of the clamps. It is now recognised that the latter technique does not really lead to high concentration of heparin in the legs but is really equivalent to systematic heparinisation with 20 mg. (10 mg. in each leg). The heparin prevents thrombosis in those arteries where blood flow has been cut off by clamping and it is reversed by injecting protamine sulphate either when the clamps have been released or at the end of the operation (p. 143).

The method of wound closure used depends on individual technique. If retroperitoneal oozing is present, a vacuum drain may be introduced and removed after 48 hours.

POST-OPERATIVE CARE

When the anaesthetist is satisfied with the patient's condition, he is transported to the recovery room where he will probably remain for 24 hours. Central venous pressure, arterial pressure, and ECG monitoring are usually continued during this period. Continuous oxygen (4 litres/minute by Edinburgh mask) is required for about 24 hours, pulse and blood pressure and urinary output should each be charted hourly. If the latter falls below an agreed level (e.g., 30 ml. per hour) mannitol (100 ml. of 20 per cent solution) should be given and repeated as necessary during the first 48 hours. Deep breathing and leg movement is actively encouraged.

The patient is nursed flat on one or two pillows for the first 48 hours. It is important to attend to pressure areas during this time, to alter the patient's position periodically, and to encourage active movements of his legs. The catheter is removed after 48 hours and he is allowed out of bed as soon as his ileus has settled. Oral fluids are restricted to 30 ml. hourly until flatus is passed freely and the naso-gastric tube is removed. The intravenous infusion is discontinued when he can take an adequate quantity of fluids orally.

Antibiotic cover is continued for seven days. Sutures are re-removed at 12 to 14 days and the patient should be fit to go home by the fifteenth day. By using strong non-absorbable sutures for the rectus sheath it is possible to allow a patient home after seven days provided home circumstances are good and he is moving about adequately.

COMPLICATIONS

There are many technical mishaps which can occur during operation leading to thrombosis of arteries or death of the patient but details of these are beyond the scope of this book.

Operative mortality. This depends to some extent on the nature and scope of the operation and on the fitness of the patient. In general, a relatively high degree of operative risk may be acceptable in cases of abdominal aneurysm or where operation is undertaken for relief of gangrene, but operative risks are unacceptable in patients with intermittent claudication. In any mixed series of cases, the operative mortality rate should be less than 5 per cent.

Principal causes of death are severe haemorrhage causing cardiac arrest, post-operative coronary thrombosis, pulmonary embolism and renal tubular necrosis. Control of *haemorrhage* is a technical matter and deaths from this cause should be rare. *Coronary thrombosis* is most liable to occur in the older or unfit patient and the selection of cases for operation plays an important part in minimising this risk. *Pulmonary embolism* is a hazard of all major operations and its incidence can be reduced by encouraging the patient to move his legs and body as soon as he recovers from the operation and by getting him out of bed as soon as possible. Even with high standards of care, however, this cause is likely to contribute 1 per cent to the mortality rate of aorto-iliac operations. *Renal tubular necrosis* is a rare cause of death provided hypotension is treated as soon as it is evident and mannitol is infused when urine secretion falls off.

Hypotension. This may occur during the first 48 hours. If the systolic blood pressure falls to 100 mm. Hg or less and the patient had a normal pressure before operation, corrective measures should be commenced immediately. The foot of the bed is elevated, blood or plasma is given and, if these do not suffice, drugs may be given to raise the pressure (e.g., cortisone, aramine). Urine output must be carefully watched as the risk of tubular necrosis is high whenever hypotension is severe or prolonged.

Paralytic ileus. A mild degree of paralytic ileus occurs in almost every case due to the peri-aortic dissection and the division of sympathetic nerve fibres. It usually settles within three to four days and oral feeding must be withheld until it does. Recovery is indicated by the return of bowel sounds, a lessening of abdominal distension, and the passage of flatus and faeces. During this time, the intravenous infusion of 2 units of 5 per cent dextrose in water alternating with 1 unit of normal saline to a daily total of 2½ to 3 litres provides a safe régime when checked by the estimation of urea and electrolytes. If intravenous fluids are required for more than three days, plasma sodium and chloride tend to fall and the proportion of saline in the intravenous fluids must be increased.

Ileus sometimes persists for 7 to 10 days and control of this situation is more difficult. Oral fluids should be strictly limited to 30 ml. hourly. After the third day, it becomes necessary to add potassium to the intravenous fluid and, as soon as there is any indication that ileus will be prolonged, additional calories should be given intravenously in the form of Aminosol, Aminosol-fructose-ethanol, fructose, or Intralipid in order that a daily intake of 2,000 to 3,000 cal. can be achieved. With patience, the ileus will settle provided that the possibility of actual intestinal obstruction has been excluded.

Intestinal obstruction. During healing, there is a great deal of inflammatory change around the operation site and a part of the small intestine, usually the terminal ileum, may become adherent and kinked. Intestinal obstruction is indicated by the development of abdominal pain, distension, vomiting and constipation, and may occur before the patient leaves hospital or subsequent to dismissal. Division of the offending adhesions is easily performed at laparotomy with complete relief of the obstruction.

Wound rupture: incisional hernia. Care must be taken when sewing up the incision because post-operative distension places a great strain on the suture line. If this gives way completely, resuture of the wound is required. If only the muscle layers of the abdominal wall give way and the skin remains intact, bowel will tend to

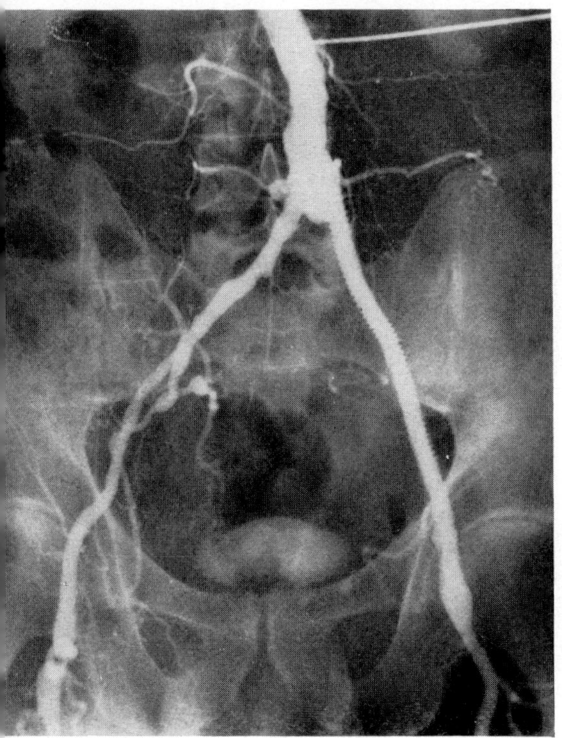

FIG. 67. Unilateral aorto-femoral bypass graft. The crimped Dacron graft has been inserted between the aorta and left common femoral artery and dye flows down into the profunda artery. This operation was successful in restoring circulation to the left leg and avoiding amputation.

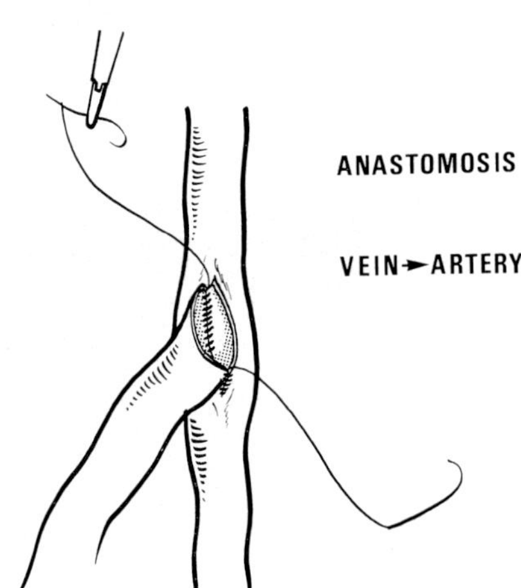

FIG. 68. Suture of the bypass vein graft to artery is partially completed.

To face page 152

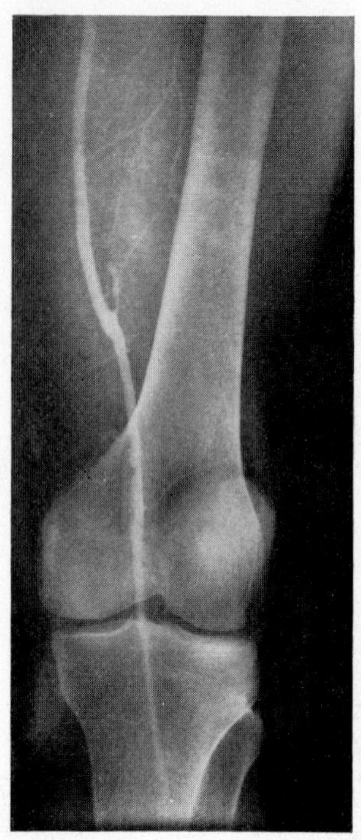

FIG. 69. Arteriogram of bypass vein graft from com
femoral artery to popliteal artery two years after op
tion. The notch on the medial side of the popliteal a
at the level of the upper pole of the patella is an ath
matous plaque which has developed since operat

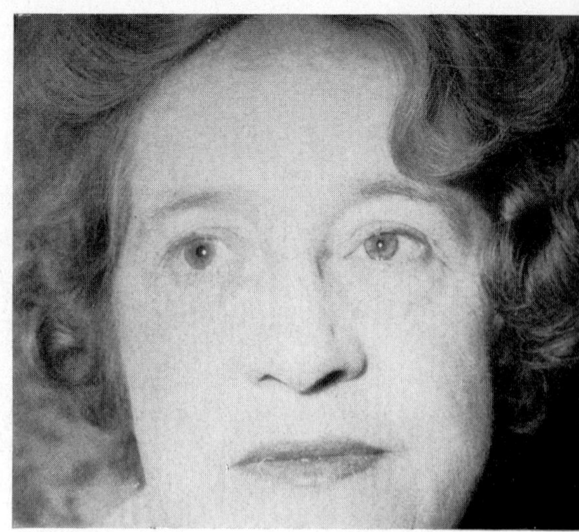

FIG. 70. Horner's syndrome: the left eye is narrower than the right and the pupil is small.

herniate through the muscle gap. The resulting incisional hernia is a large one and requires further operation or an abdominal corset to control it.

Pulmonary complications. These are surprisingly uncommon considering the length of the incision and the immobilisation in bed made necessary by the paralytic ileus. Persistent pyrexia in the first two or three days after operation indicates the need for chest X-ray and the administration of a different antibiotic pending the identification of the causative organism from sputum culture. The physiotherapist and nursing staff must encourage the patient to cough and clear the bronchi of sputum.

Pulmonary embolism. This is an uncommon cause of trouble in a well-run unit. After any operation there is an increased tendency of the blood to thrombose and this, in conjunction with the slowing down of the venous return from the legs due to recumbency, may lead to thrombosis in the calf, popliteal, femoral or iliac veins. This type of thrombus is not adherent to the vein wall and may become detached as an embolus and plug the pulmonary arteries. A small embolus will produce a lung infarct with chest pain and blood in the sputum and a large one may cause sudden death.

The best treatment is prevention and all members of staff must ensure that the patient is encouraged to move his legs freely as soon as he recovers from the anaesthetic.

Sepsis. Wound sepsis is usually superficial and unimportant. Infected wounds gradually heal and their main importance lies in their liability to cause wound rupture or incisional hernia.

On the other hand, infection involving a prosthetic graft is a serious condition leading to non-healing, separation of the graft suture line, and subsequent haemorrhage which may be fatal. Should this develop, the only possible treatment is removal of the graft and all foreign material.

The possibility of infection is increased when the patient has been in hospital for a considerable time before operation. Prevention of this complication is achieved by delaying admission of the patient until 48 hours before operation, and by giving antibiotic cover which begins before operation and stops about seven days post-operatively.

Infection caused by the staphylococcus aureus is the commonest cause of graft failure due to infection and it is possible to prevent or minimise this by giving an antibiotic whose spectrum is relatively narrow and which is effective against staphylococci. Cloxacillin (orbenin) in a dosage of 250 or 500 mg. 6-hourly has proved satisfactory in preventing graft infection and superinfection by other organisms has not been troublesome.

RESULTS

Provided that the surgeon selects his patients carefully, the results of operation are excellent. The mortality rate is below 5 per cent and the technical success rate is high.

The success of operation is measured in terms of patency rates. The early (or immediate) patency rate is the percentage of arterial reconstructions patent when the patients leave hospital. In normal circumstances, this should exceed 90 per cent. The late patency rates are usually described as 1-year patency, 5-year patency, etc. This is the percentage of patients alive with patent grafts at 1 year, 5 years, etc.

As the years go by, the patency rate declines. Grafts may thrombose for technical reasons, they may be affected by atherosclerotic changes especially at the junction of graft and artery, or the patient may die from other causes. The commonest causes of late deaths are those due to atherosclerosis elsewhere, e.g., coronary artery thrombosis or cerebro-vascular disease, but other unrelated causes such as carcinoma also affect the patency rates. A reasonably successful series of cases would show patency rates of 75 per cent at 1 year and 50 per cent at 5 years.

Case selection influences patency rates to an important degree. Operations for gangrene tend to give poorer long-term results and the older the group of patients the poorer the results are likely to be.

Femoro-popliteal Operations

PRE-OPERATIVE MANAGEMENT

The patient's fitness is assessed before admission by a careful physical examination and X-ray of chest, electrocardiogram and haemoglobin estimation are performed. Arrangements are made for 2 to 4 units of blood to be available and the patient is admitted 2 days before operation. The patient is shaved from umbilical level to ankle level on the appropriate side and the leg is thoroughly washed and prepared. An antibiotic is commenced before operation.

OPERATION

Anaesthesia is induced with pentothal then continued with the agents of the anaesthetist's choice. There are no special precautions other than the maintenance of a normal blood pressure during operation.

If a bypass femoro-popliteal vein graft is to be performed, an incision is made in the groin to expose the common femoral artery and the upper end of the long saphenous vein. The vein is dissected out of the subcutaneous tissue through one or more separate incisions along its length and the lowest incision is deepened to expose the popliteal artery above or below the level of the knee joint according to the level at which arteriography has shown the artery to be patent. The vein is lifted out and its branches are tied off with 2/0 (or finer) silk ligatures. Saline from a 20 ml. syringe is gently forced into the lower end of the vein which gradually dilates to a maximum. Any leak of saline through a previously unrecognised branch is stopped by means of a ligature or a stitch (Fig. 66).

If the vein can be distended to a reasonable diameter, the operation proceeds as planned: 50 mg. heparin are given intravenously, the popliteal artery is occluded above and below the projected site of anastomosis by clamps, and a longitudinal slit of 1 to 1½ cm. long is made in the artery. The original proximal end of saphenous vein is slit to a length matching the length of the arteriotomy and is sewn with a continuous 4/0 or 5/0 non-absorbable suture to the margin of the hole in the artery (Figs. 68 and 69). The anastomosis is tested by the release of one or more clamps and, if there is much leakage, additional interrupted sutures may be required.

A tunnel is now made either subcutaneously or below the deep fascia by means of a curved tube rather like a sigmoidoscope and the vein is threaded through and brought out in the groin. Care must be taken to avoid twisting of the vein by aligning it while it is distended with saline.

The common, superficial and deep femoral arteries are then occluded, and an incision is made in the common femoral artery. The top end of the vein graft is slit to the same length and anastomosed to the artery. The anastomosis is tested to see if additional sutures are necessary. When satisfied, the surgeon removes the distal clamps to expel air from the artery then all clamps are taken off and blood is allowed to flow down the vein. If there is any brisk bleeding, clamps are reapplied and additional sutures inserted. The heparin is then reversed and residual bleeding stops within a few minutes, either spontaneously or after lightly packing a swab over the anastomosis. If there is much oozing from the popliteal fossa, a vacuum drain is inserted and brought out through the skin below the wound. The wounds are sewn up loosely with 2/0 catgut sutures for deep fascia and subcutaneous tissues and the skin is sutured with silk. A light dressing and sometimes a loosely applied crepe bandage complete the procedure.

If the saphenous vein is too small, too varicose, or otherwise unsuitable, or if the surgeon prefers to undertake thrombo-endarterectomy, the artery is exposed through one long incision and mobilised from the accompanying vein and other structures wherever it is patent. Clamps are applied to the artery and its patent tributaries and the atheromatous material is removed by means of arterial strippers through multiple incisions in the artery. These incisions are kept to a minimum compatible with adequate removal of the intima. They may be transverse in which case simple closure of the incision by interrupted 4/0 or 5/0 sutures is all that is necessary or longitudinal when closure is effected by sewing in a patch of saphenous vein. Simple suture of a longitudinal incision would lead to narrowing of the artery and restriction of the volume of blood flow and the vein patch avoids this. The lowest incision should usually be longitudinal so that the intimal flap at the bottom of the thrombo-endarterectomy does not cause abrupt narrowing of the reconstituted artery and one or more stitches may have to be inserted to attach this flap firmly to the arterial wall in case it becomes detached and blocks the vessel.

The lower anastomosis of a bypass vein graft has no intimal flap to strip up and cause trouble and some surgeons prefer to do a thrombo-endarterectomy of the proximal part of the femoral artery and then attach a short bypass vein graft between the lower end of the rebored segment and the popliteal artery. This technique is useful when only the top 10 cm. of saphenous vein is large enough to be used as a bypass graft.

POST-OPERATIVE CARE

At the end of operation the patient usually looks pale and cold. Oxygen is given routinely and pulse and blood pressure are charted hourly. When he recovers consciousness he is instructed to move his legs.

The patient usually recovers from the effects of operation fairly quickly and appears fit and well the following day. By this time, the circulation has stabilised, ankle pulses are often palpable and the foot is warm and healthy. Special supervision is unnecessary after the initial period of recovery.

Drains are removed at 48 hours, the patient is sitting in a chair on the second post-operative day and he is able to start walking within a few days, the speed of ambulation depending largely on the extent of muscle division during operation. Sutures can be removed at 10 to 12 days and the patient allowed home soon thereafter.

COMPLICATIONS

Recovery after most femoro-popliteal operations is rapid and straightforward and the patient is usually no more upset than after an operation for hernia. The mortality rate is low (less than 1 per cent) and the only likely causes of death are coronary artery thrombosis and pulmonary embolism. However, certain specific complications do occur after this type of surgery.

Wound healing. Sometimes this is slow and extensive superficial sloughing may occur along the margin of the wound. This is caused by a number of factors: the thigh has an extensive collateral circulation before operation which is suddenly reduced when the main line flow is re-opened, the removal of the saphenous vein may impede venous return from the skin edges, there is a certain amount of drying of exposed tissue during operation and infection may be introduced. Healing of these wounds is slow but is eventually complete and the operative procedure is seldom prejudiced.

Infection. Infection involving the vein graft itself is rare and is virtually eliminated as a cause of failure by giving antibiotic cover.

Swelling. The leg is commonly swollen and this may be temporary or persistent. Its cause is obscure as venography usually shows that the deep veins are patent but where it persists for months, it is probably caused by deep vein thrombosis. Swelling is controlled by raising the foot of the bed and by applying a firm crepe bandage from toe to knee. The patient is permitted normal activity and, if the swelling persists, he is given an elastic stocking to wear when he returns home.

Pulmonary. Such complications, due to lobar collapse or to thrombo-embolism, are rare.

RESULTS

The results obtained depend to some extent on the severity of the arterial disease and the state of the distal arteries. Because of the low mortality and morbidity, operation for gangrene is worthwhile if a segmental block can be re-opened or bypassed. Many surgeons adopt an aggressive policy in such cases and expect to have a lower success rate than a more conservative surgeon. On the whole, a 50 per cent salvage rate is satisfactory and the only disadvantage of failure to achieve revascularisation is the necessity to amputate the leg at a higher level than might otherwise have been necessary, e.g., mid-thigh instead of below-knee.

Surgeons differ greatly in their attitude to intermittent claudication. As the number of patients who deteriorate and develop gangrene are few and most are still able to work in spite of claudication, most surgeons restrict operation to those patients who are severely handicapped and can walk only 50 to 100 yards. Other surgeons will operate on patients with a less severe disability and will enjoy a higher overall success rate because the arterial disease is not extensive or severe. In most series, the immediate patency rates should exceed 90 per cent. Re-thrombosis in the same leg or occlusion developing in the other leg due to extension of the athero-sclerosis are quite common and the late patency rate of the operated leg always falls off rapidly. Operation may therefore be disappointing in the long term yet it is worthwhile in a sufficiently large number of patients to justify its use in selected cases.

SYMPATHECTOMY

The smaller arteries in a limb are normally subjected to vaso-constrictor impulses originating in the sympathetic nervous system. This is a system of ganglia containing nerve cells connected by nerve fibres to form the sympathetic chain which runs down each side of the vertebral column. Removal of a segment of the chain will allow dilatation of the arteries in the part of the body supplied from that segment and there will be an increase in blood flow, mainly to the skin. Sufficient increase in flow may be obtained to relieve rest pain but improvement in claudication is uncommon except in young patients. The hand or foot becomes warmer and also dry because the sweat glands are controlled by the sympathetic nerves and no longer secrete when their nerve supply is divided.

Lumbar sympathectomy (ganglionectomy)

The leg arteries are innervated from the ganglia at the side of the lumbar spine. Removal of the lumbar sympathetic chain has no effect on atheromatous or occluded arteries but does allow dilatation of the collateral vessels.

OPERATION

The patient is anaesthetised and is placed in the supine or semi-lateral position on the operating table. An oblique or transverse incision is made in the loin and the peritoneum is pushed medially without opening it. The psoas muscle on the posterior abdominal wall is exposed and the sympathetic chain is sought at the side of the vertebral column just in front of the attachment of the psoas muscle and behind either the aorta or inferior vena cava. The chain is identified from its ganglionic swellings and is removed as far upwards and downwards as is reasonably possible, care being taken to avoid damaging the thin-walled lumbar veins which run across or behind it. When bleeding is controlled, the wound is closed with or without suction drainage.

Post-operative convalescence is rarely a problem and the patient can go home in 10 days time—or earlier.

The only common complications are haemorrhage and ileus. Haemorrhage and haematoma formation are avoided by meticulous haemostasis and the use of drainage where necessary. Paralytic ileus is unlikely when operation is unilateral but, if both lumbar chains are removed at the same time, a moderate degree of ileus may appear due to interference with the sympathetic innervation of bowel. Severe cases may require treatment by gastric suction and intravenous fluids until the bowel resumes normal activity.

Upper thoracic sympathectomy (cervical sympathectomy)

The sympathetic nerve supply to the arm vessels arises from the upper thoracic segments of the spinal cord via the upper thoracic ganglia. The immediate effect of operation is to increase blood supply to the hand and arm which becomes warm and dry but, as the years go by, some degree of sympathetic control is re-established and the effects of the operation tend to wear off. For this reason, operation is usually withheld until symptoms are severe or until tissue necrosis develops.

The second and third thoracic ganglia and related nerve chain are removed but the first or stellate ganglion is left intact. Removal of this or any of the cervical ganglia will give rise to Horner's syndrome (retraction of the eye, constriction of the pupil and drooping of the upper eyelid), and female patients especially may complain if this should result (Fig. 70).

The upper thoracic ganglia may be approached from above the clavicle—the cervical approach; through the chest—the axillary approach; or by resection of the necks of the ribs—the posterior approach. The axillary approach between the second and third ribs is probably the best except that, when the surgeon also wishes to explore the subclavian artery, the cervical approach is preferable.

Phenol Injection of the Sympathetic Chain

As an alternative to sympathectomy, the sympathetic chain can be injected with 1:15 phenol in water. This destroys the nerve fibres and results in an improvement in circulation equivalent to that of surgical sympathectomy. Provided the operator is prepared to spend time in acquiring the necessary skill, the results are satisfactory and the method has the advantage of being applicable to patients who are unfit for any operative procedure.

Other Operations for Intermittent Claudication

When it is impossible to improve the blood supply to the calf muscles, it is sometimes possible to improve the claudication distance of a patient by reducing the bulk of the calf muscles or the amount of work they have to perform. This may be done by dividing the Achilles tendon—Achilles tenotomy; by dividing the nerve supply to the calf muscles—popliteal neurectomy; or by crushing their nerve supply—selective nerve crush.

None of these operations is used routinely but they have a definite value in selected cases.

Amputations

Amputation is, unfortunately, the eventual sequel in many patients who develop gangrene due to emboli, extensive or multiple arterial occlusions, or progressive arterial occlusion. It is more common in extensive popliteal and tibial occlusions than with lesions elsewhere and it is often required in diabetes mellitus because of spreading infection. In many elderly patients, it is a terminal event, symptomatic of progressive cardio-vascular degeneration.

Amputation should never be regarded as the ultimate disablement, because many amputees of all ages adapt themselves to their disability and resume more or less normal activity.

The decision to amputate is made when gangrene has extended on to the dorsum of the foot, when ischaemic rest pain is intolerable and the patient's general condition deteriorates from lack of sleep, and when infection cannot be controlled by antibiotics. It is sometimes possible to avert or limit the extent of amputation by reconstructive surgery or sympathectomy but, in many cases, an early decision to amputate will save the patient from prolonged misery.

Amputation of the toes is seldom possible in atherosclerotic patients but may be possible in thrombo-angiitis obliterans. Transmetatarsal amputation can sometimes be achieved when the arterial disease is peripheral, but the choice is usually between below-knee, through-knee or above-knee amputations. Of these three, below-knee amputation gives the least disability, because the introduction of the patellar bearing artificial limb dispenses with cumbersome thigh straps and hinges and gives the patient a reasonable degree of mobility. The judicious use of sympathectomy or sympathetic block together with the formation of a long posterior flap whose nourishment is better than the anterior flap may enable the surgeon to obtain a healed 4 in. below-knee stump.

The next best choice is a through-knee amputation or a Gritti-Stokes amputation in which the articular surface of the patella is removed and the raw surface is applied to the lower end of the femur whose articular surface has also been removed.

So far as possible, the surgeon should amputate at a level which will ensure primary healing and, unfortunately, this is often only possible at mid-thigh. A minority of patients become bilateral amputees, the second leg being amputated a year or two after the first and, in general, both amputations should be at the same level.

APPENDIX A

Common ECG Patterns

Cardiac arrhythmias are common during the first few days after cardiac surgery. They may be caused by the exposure and handling of the heart which is necessary in every operation, interference with the conduction pathways during certain operations or hypoxia and electrolyte imbalance. Some types of arrhythmia are of little significance and do not affect the patient's post-operative progress. Others may produce a reduction in cardiac output which leads to a fall in coronary blood flow and further myocardial impairment. When this occurs, recovery may be impossible and the onset of arryhthmia may commence a sequence of events which leads to death of the patient.

The ECG should be monitored for at least 24 hours after major heart surgery so that arrhythmias can be detected as soon as they develop and the correct treatment instituted. It is therefore important that the trained nurse should be able to recognise the normal ECG and the common abnormalities in order that early treatment can be instituted.

Sinus rhythm (normal)

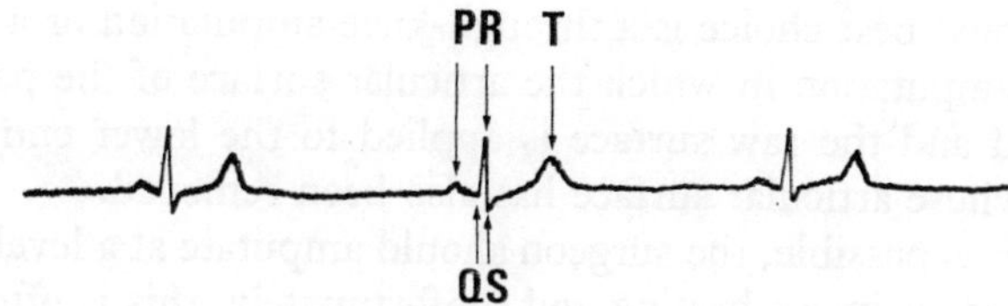

FIG. 71. Normal sinus rhythm.

Each normal heart beat is accompanied by five spikes or waves on the ECG tracing.

The P wave occurs with contraction of the atria.

The Q, R and S waves denote contraction of the ventricles.

The T wave occurs when the ventricles are relaxed.

Left ventricular hypertrophy (LVH)

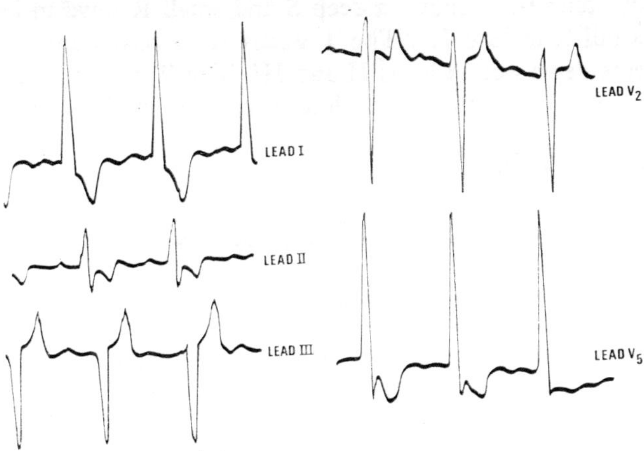

FIG. 72. Left ventricular hypertrophy.

The record is from a patient with aortic valve disease. It shows an abnormally high R wave in Lead I and V5, and an abnormally deep S wave in lead III and V2. The ST segment is depressed in V5.

Right ventricular hypertrophy (RVH)

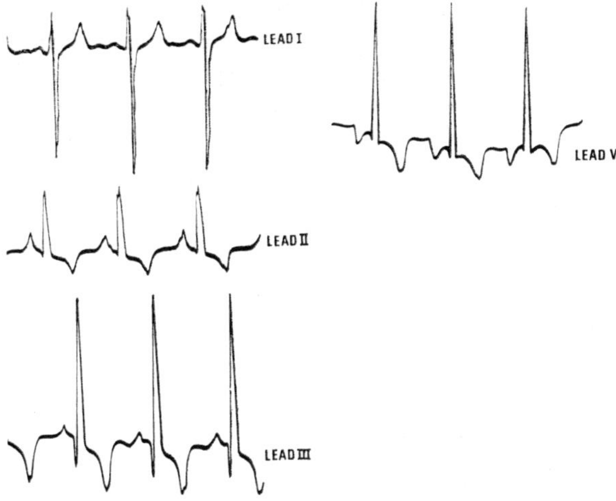

FIG. 73. Right ventricular hypertrophy.

The record is from a patient with an atrial septal defect and pulmonary stenosis. It shows a deep S and small R wave in lead I, with a tall R in lead III. The T waves are inverted and the ST segments depressed in leads II and III. The R wave is tall in V1 and the S wave is absent. The downward wave in V1 is a Q wave.

Auricular fibrillation

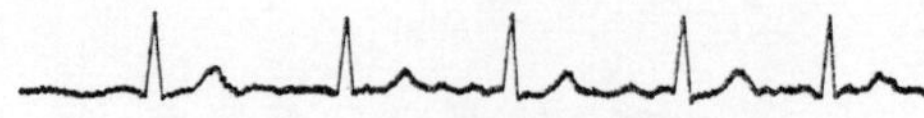

FIG. 74. Auricular fibrillation.

In this condition, the atrium contracts irregularly so that the P waves are absent and are replaced by a number of small ripples. Electrical stimuli reach the ventricle at irregular intervals so that the QRST complexes are spaced irregularly.

Auricular fibrillation is not usually a dangerous arrythmia. It should be suspected if the heart rate suddenly becomes fast and irregular. Some of the ventricular contractions are too feeble to transmit a pulse wave to the radial artery, so that the number of beats counted at the apex is greater than that counted at the wrist. The difference between the apex rate and pulse rate is called a pulse deficit. If it exceeds 20/minute, the blood pressure falls and the patient's general condition is likely to deteriorate. Treatment consists of giving digoxin, either orally or intravenously, which slows the apex rate and increases the force of cardiac contraction. Alternatively, when fibrillation is of recent onset, quinidine or electrical cardioversion using the defibrillator may restore normal rhythm.

Auricular flutter

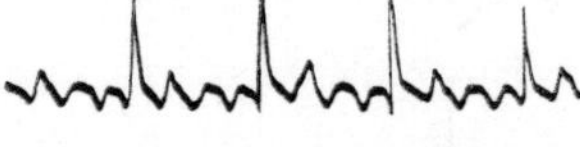

FIG. 75. Auricular flutter.

In this condition, the atria beat regularly at very fast rates (more than 250/minute). The A-V node cannot transmit impulses as fast as this and the ventricles respond to only every second or third atrial beat. Accordingly, the ECG tracing shows two or three P waves for every QRST complex. Treatment again consists of the use of digoxin, electrical cardioversion or quinidine.

Ventricular extra-systoles (ventricular ectopic beats)

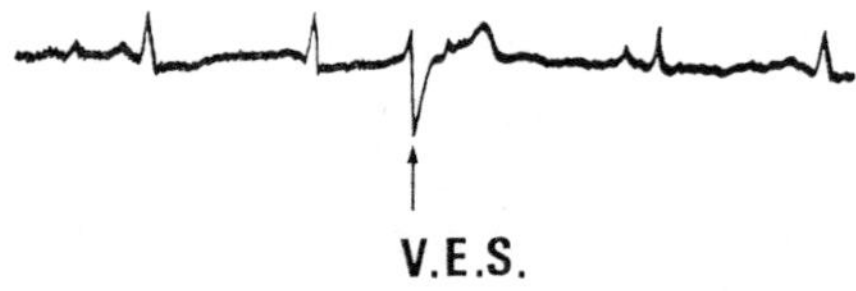

FIG. 76. Ventricular extra-systole.

This arrhythmia is recognised on the ECG tracing as a widened QRS complex followed by a pause before the next normal beat.

The common causes are (1) mechanical irritation of the ventricles (e.g., by a catheter or a pericardial drain), (2) digoxin overdosage, (3) hypokalaemia (low serum potassium level), (4) hypoxia.

Occasional ventricular extra-systoles are very common after cardiac surgery due to the handling and disturbance of the heart. If they are more frequent than 10/minute, their frequency should be charted and treatment instituted.

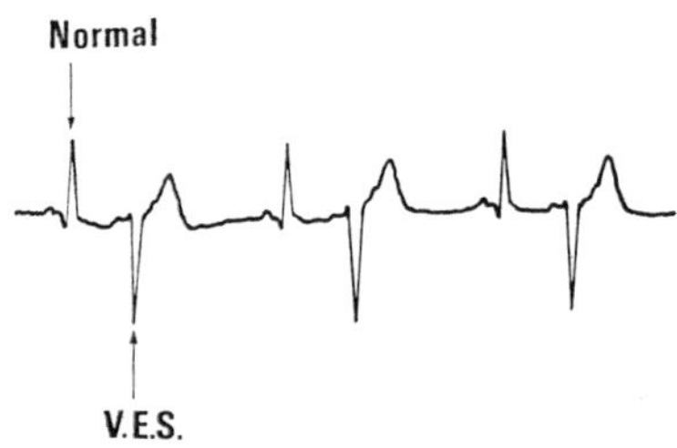

FIG. 77. Coupled beats.

Figure 77. When every second beat is an extra-systole, two beats occur together followed by a pause, and this is called 'coupling'. This may be due to digoxin overdosage, but otherwise it may prove to be a serious arrhythmia.

Groups of ventricular extra-systoles have an ominous significance and often precede ventricular tachycardia or ventricular fibrillation which are extremely serious. Urgent treatment is required.

TREATMENT

1. Stop digoxin dosage if it is suspected that this is the cause of extra-systoles.

2. Check plasma potassium level.

3. Procaine amide (100 mg./minute) can be given intravenously to a total of 1·0 g. This is maintained by a slow drip of 1 to 2 g. in 500 ml. 5 per cent dextrose in water.

N.B. Procaine amide lowers the blood pressure and should only be given where the blood pressure can be monitored frequently.

4. Lignocaine (1·0 to 2·0 mg./kg. body weight) can be given slowly intravenously. This is maintained by a slow i.v. drip of 1·0 g. in 500 ml. 5 per cent dextrose in water. Lignocaine should be given via a 'paediatric' drip set so that inadvertent overdosage will be less likely. An i.v. drip containing lignocaine should not be left unattended.

N.B. Lignocaine may lower the blood pressure or cause respiratory arrest and convulsions and it must therefore be used with care.

Ventricular tachycardia

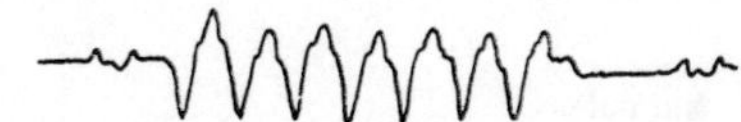

FIG. 78. Paroxysmal ventricular tachycardia.

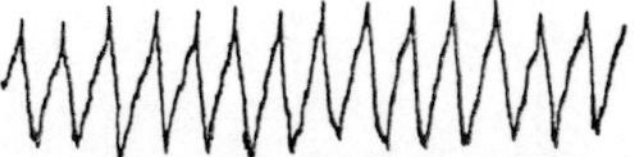

FIG. 79. Ventricular tachycardia (or flutter).

In this condition, ventricular ectopic beats occur in rapid regular succession and the ECG shows a 'saw-tooth' pattern. This type of arrhythmia is dangerous and is associated with a fall in blood pressure and a rise in central venous pressure. Treatment is required urgently because the heart is beating very inefficiently and the prognosis is grave.

Treatment by electrical cardioversion, procaine amide, or lignocaine may restore normal rhythm.

Ventricular fibrillation (VF)

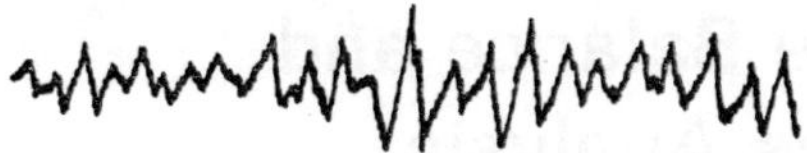

FIG. 80. Ventricular fibrillation.

When ventricular fibrillation occurs, there is no ventricular contraction and cardiac output stops. The circulation ceases, the blood pressure falls to zero and unconsciousness follows in a few seconds.

Irreversible brain damage occurs within about three minutes, and unless immediate effective action is taken by those at the bedside, the patient will die. Immediate external cardiac massage must be commenced until a defibrillator can be brought into use. Other measures required in circulatory arrest are the administration of 200 mEq of sodium bicarbonate intravenously to correct the metabolic acidosis, the induction of a diuresis with mannitol (20 g. in 100 ml. i.v.), and the administration of oxygen.

APPENDIX B

Acid-base Balance and Blood Gas Analysis

The normal hydrogen ion concentration of the blood (pH) is maintained within very narrow limits by the balanced interaction of acids and alkalis. Acids are produced continuously by the tissues during the metabolisation of carbohdyrate and fat to produce energy. These acids are neutralised by several mechanisms, of which the most important is the bicarbonate store of the body. The chemical interaction between the acid products of metabolism and the bicarbonate stores produces salts (which are excreted in the urine) and carbon dioxide (which is excreted by the lungs).

Myocardial function is very sensitive to changes in the acid-base balance of the blood and careful monitoring of this balance is an important part of the management of cardiac surgical patients.

The three measurements used to assess the acid-base status of the patient are the pH, the carbon dioxide content of the blood (P_{CO_2}) and the bicarbonate content of the blood ('standard bicarbonate'). These three parameters are measured from capillary or arterial blood samples and the normal values are:

pH — 7·4
P_{CO_2} — 40 mm. Hg
St. Bic. — 24 mEq./litre

The abnormal states which may develop after cardiac surgery are as follows:

RESPIRATORY ACIDOSIS

This is due to inadequate ventilation and is seen most commonly in patients whose breathing is too shallow or too infrequent because of wound pain.

It results in an excess of carbon dioxide in the blood, and typical acid-base figures from a patient with respiratory acidosis would be:

pH — 7·25 (low)
P_{CO_2} — 80 mm. Hg (raised)
St. Bic. — 24 mEq/litre (normal)

The first step in treatment is to encourage deep breathing. Analgesics given in sufficient dosage to relieve pain without depressing respiration can be used, and the physiotherapist encourages the patient with breathing exercises. If this fails to reduce the arterial P_{CO_2}, mechanical ventilation may be required.

METABOLIC ACIDOSIS

This condition is due to an accumulation of acid products during abnormal metabolism. In cardiac surgical patients, it is a consequence of a low cardiac output and/or peripheral vasoconstriction. These conditions cause tissue hypoxia and, in the absence of an adequate supply of oxygen, the tissues release acids. These acids are neutralised by the bicarbonate stores which gradually become depleted.

Typical acid-base figures in an arterial sample would be:

pH — 7·2 (low)
P_{CO_2} — 40 mm. Hg (normal)
St. Bic. — 18 mEq./litre (low)

Treatment consists of the intravenous administration of sodium bicarbonate in a dose calculated to restore the bicarbonate stores to normal (dose in mEq. = base deficit $\times \frac{1}{3}$ body wt. in kg.). However, this treatment will only succeed when the cause of the metabolic acidosis can be corrected, e.g., increasing the supply of oxygen to the tissues by administering oxygen and correcting the low cardiac output and/or vasoconstriction.

METABOLIC ALKALOSIS

Progressive metabolic alkalosis develops during the first post-operative week in many patients who have undergone open-heart surgery. Several factors contribute to the development of this condition, but the principal factor is the volume of blood transfused. Donor blood is preserved by a citrate-dextrose compound which is metabolised by the body with the production of sodium bicarbonate.

Typical figures are:

pH — 7·5 (high)
P_{CO_2} — 45 mm. Hg (high)
St. Bic. — 30 mEq./litre (high)

Treatment is rarely required, but excess bicarbonate in the tissue fluids and blood can cause a reduction in plasma potassium levels and potassium supplements may be necessary.

Arterial oxygen measurements (P_{O_2} levels)

Hypoxia is one of the most dangerous situations which can develop after major surgery and careful monitoring of the oxygen content of arterial blood is an essential part of the post-operative management of cardiac surgical patients.

Patients with heart disease usually have an associated abnormality of lung function which is further impaired by anaesthesia and heart-lung bypass. Hypoxia tends to develop post-operatively and the oxygen concentration of the air breathed by patients is increased by administering oxygen for the first few days. The amount of oxygen required is determined by measurement of the oxygen content of arterial blood samples.

The amount of oxygen in a blood sample is measured in terms of its pressure or 'tension' in millimetres of mercury—P_{O_2}. When a person with normal heart and lungs breathes air, the arterial P_{O_2} is 80 mm. Hg; when a normal person breathes pure oxygen, the arterial P_{O_2} will be about 400 mm. Hg. (Air is a mixture of one-fifth oxygen and four-fifths nitrogen.)

After thoracotomy and cardiac surgery, the oxygen transferring function of the lungs is impaired and the oxygen content of arterial blood may become dangerously low, e.g., less than 60 mm. Hg. It is routine practice to administer oxygen in the post-operative period with the aim of maintaining arterial oxygen tension at a safe level. The arterial P_{O_2} usually aimed at is 120 mm. Hg. This is done by enriching the air breathed by the patient with oxygen, using some form of plastic face mask (e.g., the Edinburgh mask). The concentration of oxygen in the inspired air can be adjusted by varying the rate of oxygen flow to the mask and by adding tubular plastic extensions to the mask.

Index

ROBERT CUNNINGHAM & SONS LTD., ALVA